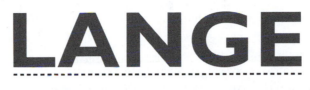

LANGE
SMART CHARTS

PHARMACOLOGY

Catherine E. Pelletier, MD

Department of Emergency Medicine
Drexel College of Medicine
Philadelphia, Pennsylvania

LANGE MEDICAL BOOKS / MCGRAW-HILL
Medical Publishing Division

New York   Chicago   San Francisco   Lisbon   London   Madrid   Mexico City
Milan   New Delhi   San Juan   Seoul   Singapore
Sydney   Toronto

D0220890

Lange Smart Charts: Pharmacology

Copyright © 2003 by The **McGraw-Hill Companies**, Inc. All rights reserved.
Printed in the United States of America. Except as permitted under the United States
Copyright Act of 1976, no part of this publication may be reproduced or distributed
in any form or by any means, or stored in a data base or retrieval system, without the
prior written permission of the publisher.

1 2 3 4 5 6 7 8 9 0 KGP/KGP 0 9 8 7 6 5 4 3

ISBN 0-07-138878-8
ISSN 1542-6866

This book was set in Goudy by TechBooks.
The editors were Janet Foltin, Harriet Lebowitz, and Nicky Panton.
The production supervisor was Philip Galea.
The art manager was Charissa Baker.
The cover designer was Mary McKeon.
The index was prepared by Jerry Ralya.

Quebecor/Kingsport was the printer and binder.

This book is printed on acid-free paper.

NOTICE

To my mother and father.
Words cannot express the depth of my love and gratitude.

CONTENTS

PREFACE

Lange Smart Charts: Pharmacology is written specifically for students in the field of medicine. The book not only highlights the information that students need to learn for course examinations and for the pharmacology component of the USMLE Step 1 boards, but also makes it easier to study and remember this material.

The unique approach of this book is immediately apparent. **Tables** and **diagrams** are used exclusively to present well-selected information clearly and concisely. This chart method gives an instant picture of how the various facts are connected, thereby making study time productive and successful. The special feature **Terms to Learn** introduces each chapter and provides the reader with the minimum essentials needed for a quick understanding of the high-yield facts–the information most often targeted on examinations and boards. **Mnemonics** are also included throughout the book to make immediate recall easier.

The material presented in *Pharmacology Smart Charts* is detailed enough for review in pharmacology courses, yet concise enough for board review. The selection and organization of information is designed to promote efficient use of study time by reducing the amount of re-reading required to master this subject area.

Special thanks to Dr. Andrea Waingold for her revisions of the anesthesia medications table and to Dr. Vivek Reddy who created the summary table on page 231. Also, thanks to Dr. Mohamed Dattu for his unending patience and support during the completion of this project.

HOW TO USE THIS BOOK

Layout of the book	The book is composed entirely of tables and diagrams to facilitate comparison and clarify relationships among drugs, drug classes, and drug mechanisms.
Using *Lange Smart Charts: Pharmacology* in conjunction with your pharmacology course	For optimal benefit, start using this book early in the year to follow along with the content of your pharmacology course. *Lange Smart Charts: Pharmacology* is designed to make the most of your studying time. Each chapter is introduced by an **outline** of the classes of drugs that are the focus of study. This is followed by **Terms to Learn,** which provides an understanding of drug classification, the pharmacodynamics and pharmacokinetics of drugs, and relevant diseases. **Diagrams** of drug categories allow quick memorization and **illustrations** clarify difficult concepts. **Tables** make it easy to associate the drugs and drug categories with the relevant high-yield facts that appear most often on the boards and on pharmacology examinations, including pharmacokinetics, mechanisms of action and resistance, clinical uses, and side effects. **Mnemonics** and other learning aids in each chapter promote quick recall of details.
Using *Lange Smart Charts: Pharmacology* as a pharmacology review for the USMLE Step 1.	Begin by reviewing each of the chapter outlines, the Terms to Learn, and the drug classification diagrams. Use the tables to fill in the details. Learn the mnemonics to improve your recall. Find your weaknesses by using a pharmacology question book and then review these topics in the relevant chapters. With this approach, you should be able to review pharmacology in a matter of days.

ABBREVIATIONS

A

AC Adenylate cyclase
ACE Angiotensin-converting enzyme
Ach Acetylcholine
ACTH Adrenocorticotropic hormone
ADH Antidiuretic hormone
ADHD Attention-deficit hyperactivity disorder
ADP Adenosine diphosphate
ANS Autonomic nervous system
AP Action potential
ATP Adenosine triphosphate
ATPase Adenosine triphosphatase
AV Atrioventricular

B

BBB Blood brain barrier
BP Blood pressure
BPH Benign prostatic hypertrophy
BMT Bone marrow transplant

C

CA Cancer
CAD Coronary artery disease
cAMP Cyclic adenosine monophosphate
CF Cystic fibrosis
cGMP Cyclic guanosine monophosphate

CHF Congestive heart failure
CMV Cytomegalovirus
CNS Central nervous system
CO Cardiac output
COMT Catechol-*o*-methyltransferase
COPD Chronic obstructive pulmonary disease
COX Cyclooxygenase
CPR Cardiopulmonary resuscitation
CRH Corticotropin-releasing hormone
CSF Cerebrospinal fluid
CTZ Chemoreceptor trigger zone
CV Cardiovascular
CVA Cerebrovascular accident
CVS Cardiovascular system

D

DA Dopamine
DAG Diacylglycerol

E

EC Extracellular
ECF Extracellular fluid
EEG Electroencephalogram
ENT Ear, nose, and throat
EPI Epinephrine
EPS Extrapyramidal side effects

F

FDA Food and Drug Administration

G

G+ Gram-positive
G− Gram-negative
G6PD Glucose-6-phosphate dehydrogenase
GERD Gastroesophageal reflux disease
GFR Glomerular filtration rate
GI Gastrointestinal
GTP Guanosine triphosphate
GU Genitourinary

H

5-HT Serotonin
Hb Hemoglobin
HDL High-density lipoprotein
HIV Human immunodeficiency virus
HMG-CoA Hepatic hydroxymethylglutaryl coenzyme A
HR Heart rate
HSV Herpes simplex virus

I

IBD Inflammatory bowel disease
IC Intracellular
IDDM Insulin dependent diabetes mellitus
IL Interleukin
IM Intramuscular
IP₃ Inositol 1, 4, 5-triphosphate
ISA Intrinsic sympathomimetic activity
IV Intravenous

L

LDL Low-density lipoprotein
LFT Liver function tests
Lp(a) Lipoprotein little A antigen
LTU Long-term use

M

MI Myocardial infarction
MAO Monoamine oxidase
MOA Mechanism of action
MRSA Methicillin-resistant *Staphylococcus aureus*
MSA Membrane stabilizing activity

N

nAch Nicotinic acetylcholine receptors
NE Norepinephrine
NIDDM Non–insulin dependent diabetes mellitus
NM Neuromuscular
NMJ Neuromuscular junction
NO Nitrous oxide
NRTI Nucleoside reverse transcriptase inhibitor
NSAID Nonsteroidal anti-inflammatory drug
NT Neurotransmitter

O

OA Osteoarthritis
OR Operating room
OTC Over the counter

P

PABA Para-aminobenzoic acid
PCP *Pneumocystis carinii* pneumonia

PDE Phosphodiesterase
PID Pelvic inflammatory disease
pK$_a$ Negative logarithm of acid ionization constant
PO Oral administration
PTT Partial thromboplastin time
PUD Peptic ulcer disease
PVD Peripheral vascular disease

R

RA Rheumatoid arthritis
RAS Reticular activating system
REM Rapid eye movement
RTA Renal tubular acidosis

S

SA Sinoatrial
SC Subcutaneous
SIADH Syndrome of inappropriate antidiuretic hormone (secretion)
SLE Systemic lupus erythematosus
SOA Site of action
SSRI Selective serotonin reuptake inhibitor

T

TB Tuberculosis
TCA Tricyclic antidepressant
TG Triglyceride

THC Tetrahydrocannabinol
TIA Transient ischemic attack
TNF Tumor necrosis factor
TPR Total peripheral resistance

U

URI Upper respiratory infection
USMLE United States Medical Licensing Examination
UTI Urinary tract infection

V

VLDL Very low-density lipoprotein
VZV Varicella-zoster virus

PHARMACOKINETICS ABBREVIATIONS:

A: Administration or Absorption
B: Biotransformation or plasma protein binding
D: Distribution
DOA: Duration of action
E: Excretion
M: Metabolism
OOA: Onset of action
R: Redistribution
$t^1\!/_2$**:** Half-life

CHAPTER 1
PHARMACOLOGY BASICS

I. PHARMACODYNAMICS

Dose-Response Curves

Comparison of Dose-Response Curves

Response Curves: Agonists and Antagonists

II. PHARMACOKINETICS

Drug Movement within the Body

Drug Solubility

Administration

Distribution and Binding

Metabolism

Elimination

Important Equations

Therapeutic Values

Dosing

TERMS TO LEARN

Agonist	A drug that activates its receptor upon binding.
Bioavailability	The percentage of administered dose that reaches the systemic circulation.
Chemical Antagonist	A drug that counters the effects of another by binding the drug and preventing its action.
Competitive Antagonist	A pharmacologic antagonist that can be overcome by increasing the dose of agonist.
EC_{50}	In graded dose-response curves, the concentration or dose that produces 50% of the maximum possible response; in quantal dose-response curves, the dose that causes the specified response in 50% of the population.
ED_{50}	Dose required to produce the desired effect in 50% of subjects.
Effector	Component of the biologic system that accomplishes the biologic effect after being activated by the receptor; often a channel or enzyme.
Efficacy	The maximum effect a drug can bring about, regardless of dose.
Graded Dose-Response Curve	A graph of the increasing responses to increasing doses of a drug.
Inert Binding Site	A component of the biologic system to which a drug binds without changing any function.
Irreversible Antagonist	A pharmacologic antagonist that cannot be overcome by increasing the dose of the agonist.
K_d	The concentration of drug that results in binding to 50% of the receptors.
LD_{50}	Dose that is lethal to 50% of subjects.
Partial Agonist	A drug that binds to its receptor but produces a smaller effect at full dosage than a full agonist.
pH	Inverse log of the hydrogen ion concentration, denotes the acidity or alkalinity of a substance.
Pharmacodynamics	The actions of the drug on the body.
Pharmacokinetics	The action of the body on the drug.
Pharmacologic Antagonist	A drug that binds to its receptor without activating it.

Pharmacology	The study of substances that interact with living systems through chemical reactions.
Physiologic Antagonist	A drug that counters the effects of another by binding to a different receptor and causing opposing effects.
pK$_a$	Inverse log of the ionization constant of an acid.
Potency	The dose or concentration required to bring about 50% of a drug's maximal effect.
Quantal Dose-Response Curve	A graph of the fraction of a population that shows a specified response to increasing doses of a drug.
Receptor	A component of the biologic system to which a drug binds to bring about a change in function of the system.
Receptor Site	The specific region of the receptor molecule at which the drug binds.
Spare Receptors	Receptors that do not have to bind drug in order for the maximum effect to be produced; ie, K_d greater than the EC$_{50}$; thought to exist if the maximal response is obtained at less than maximal receptor occupation levels.
TI$_{50}$	Drug dose that indicates the ratio of desired to undesired effects.

I. Pharmacodynamics

DOSE-RESPONSE CURVES

Type of Curve	Characteristics
Graded dose-response curve	• Unit and time are constant • Dose and effect are variable
Quantal dose-response curve	• Effect and time are constant • Dose and unit are variable • Yields safety information
Time action dose-response curve	• Unit is constant (ie, the same patient is used) • Dose, time, and effect are variable • Yields the time of onset of the action of the drug, the peak effect of the drug, and the duration of effect of the drug

COMPARISON OF DOSE-RESPONSE CURVES

Dose-Response Curve	Unit	Dose	Time	Effect
Graded	Constant	Variable	Constant	Constant
Quantal	Variable	Variable	Constant	Constant
Time Action	Constant	Variable	Variable	Variable

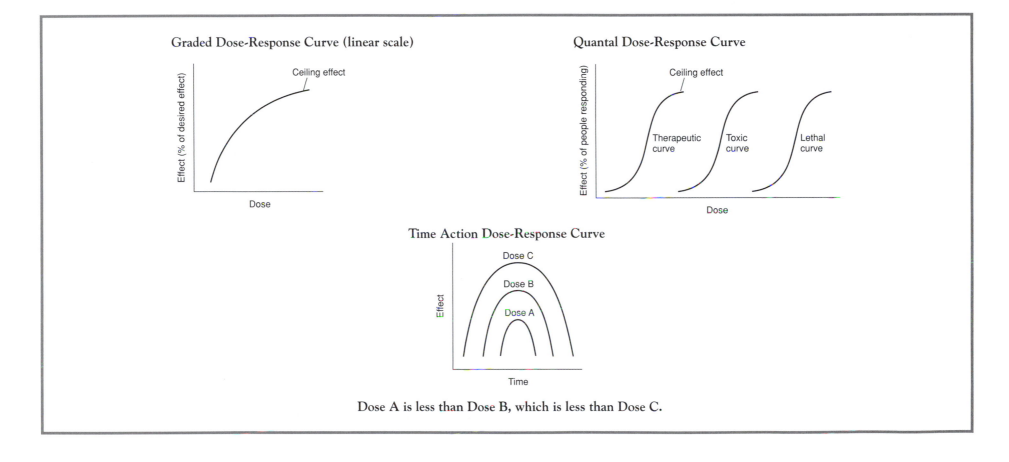

Graded Dose-Response Curve (linear scale)

Quantal Dose-Response Curve

Time Action Dose-Response Curve

Dose A is less than Dose B, which is less than Dose C.

RESPONSE CURVES: AGONISTS AND ANTAGONISTS

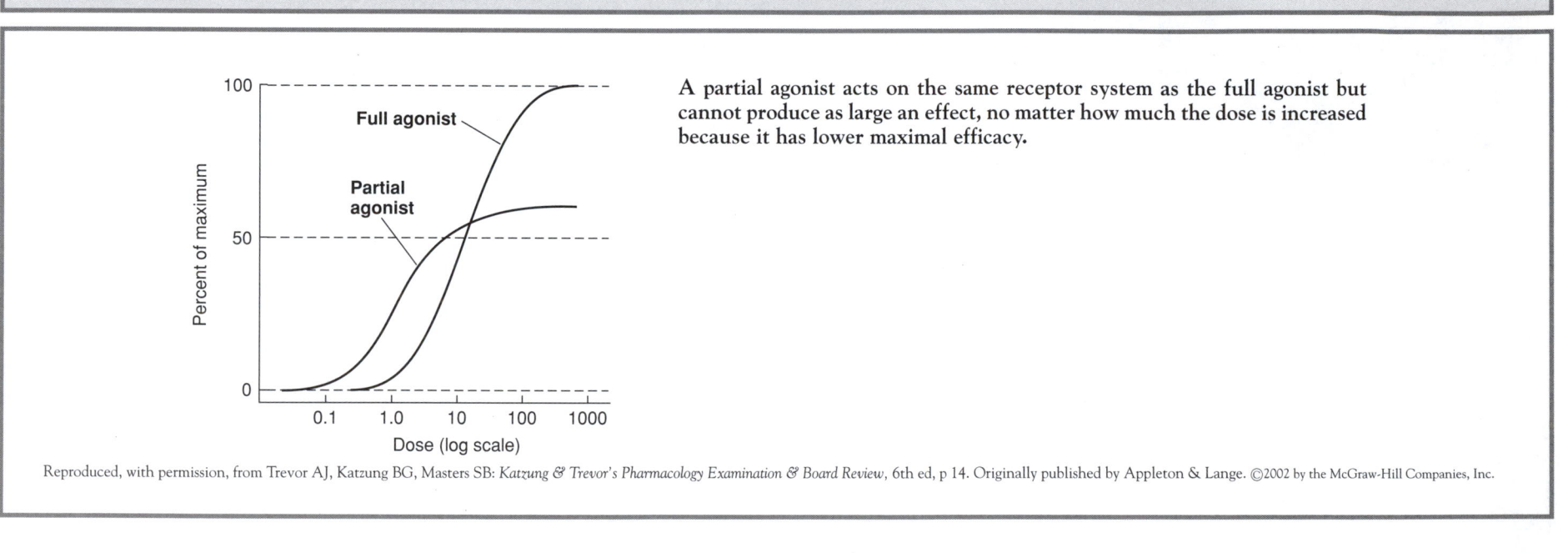

A partial agonist acts on the same receptor system as the full agonist but cannot produce as large an effect, no matter how much the dose is increased because it has lower maximal efficacy.

A competitive agonist shifts the agonist curve to the right (A); an irreversible antagonist shifts the agonist curve downward (B).

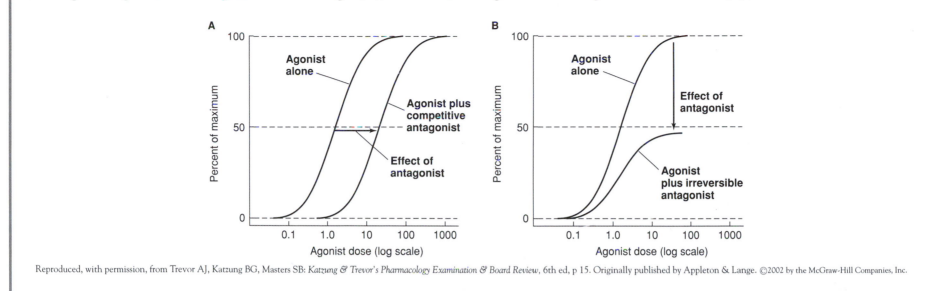

II. Pharmacokinetics

DRUG MOVEMENT WITHIN THE BODY

Type of Movement	Requirements
Passive diffusion	Requires no energy
Facilitated diffusion	Requires specific transport mechanisms; no energy required
Active transport	Links energy consuming movement of substances to energy producing mechanisms.

DRUG SOLUBILITY

- The movement of a drug within the body depends on the ionization state of the drug molecule. The Henderson-Hasselbalch equation can be used to determine the ionization state of a molecule at a specific pH:

$$pH = pK_a + \log \frac{\text{unprotonated form}}{\text{protonated form}}$$

- Aqueous solubility of a drug is proportional to the molecule's charge.
- Lipid solubility is *inversely* proportional to a molecule's charge.
- The pK_a value is specific to each molecule.

ADMINISTRATION

Route	Significant Features
Oral (PO)	Convenient; subject to first-pass metabolism by liver, which alters bioavailability
Intravenous (IV)	Rapid; 100% bioavailability
Intramuscular (IM)	Allows for larger amounts to be administered; higher bioavailability than PO; avoids first-pass metabolism
Subcutaneous (SC)	Slower absorption than IM; larger volumes of administration not possible
Buccal	Between the cheeks and gums; absorption without first-pass metabolism
Sublingual	Below the tongue; absorption without first-pass metabolism
Rectal	Less first-pass metabolism than PO administration
Inhalation	Allows for drug delivery directly to respiratory tissues; allows for rapid absorption due to large surface area of alveoli
Topical	Method of administration for local effect; slowest absorption rate
Transdermal	Skin application to achieve systemic effects

DISTRIBUTION AND BINDING

Distribution of a drug is determined by several factors:

- Blood flow to the organ
- The solubility of a drug
- The level of binding of drug (ie, to proteins within the blood)

Inert binding sites are locations on endogenous molecules that bind a drug, yielding no resultant effects. Examples of such binding sites include the plasma binding proteins, albumin, and α_1-acid glycoprotein.

METABOLISM

Functions	• Terminate drug activity • Activate drug activity (in which case, the drug administered is termed a prodrug)
Metabolic Reactions Phase 1	• Reactions that convert the parent drug to a more polar or reactive product • Reactions include: oxidation, reduction, deamination, and hydrolysis
Phase 2	• Conjugation reactions that link a polar group to the drug molecule to increase its water solubility • Polar moieties include glucuronate, acetate, glutathione, glycine, sulfate, and methyl
Sites of Metabolism	• Most drugs are metabolized by the liver. • The kidneys are another important site of metabolism. • The enzymes of degradation for a small number of drugs are spread widely throughout other tissues, including the blood and the wall of the GI tract.

ELIMINATION

Elimination determines the duration of action for most drugs, and it may take two forms:

- First order—The rate of elimination is proportional to the drug concentration, resulting in a constant half-life of elimination.
- Zero order—The rate of elimination is constant regardless of drug concentration, and the plasma concentration of the drug decreases linearly.

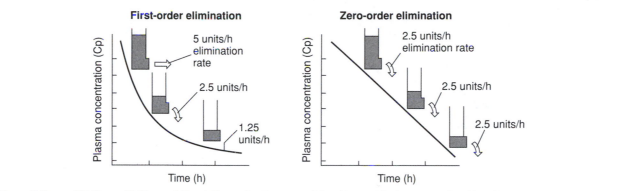

Reproduced, with permission from Trevor AJ, Katzung BG, Masters SB: *Katzung & Trevor's Pharmacology Examination & Board Review*, 6th ed, p 6. Originally published by Appleton & Lange. ©2002 by the McGraw-Hill Companies, Inc.

IMPORTANT EQUATIONS

Determination	Description	Equation
Clearance (CL)	Relates the rate of elimination to the concentration of drug within the plasma	$CL = \dfrac{\text{Rate of elimination of a drug}}{\text{Plasma concentration of the drug}}$
Volume of distribution (V_d):	Relates the amount of drug in the body to the concentration of drug in the plasma	$V_d = \dfrac{\text{Amount of drug in the body}}{\text{Plasma concentration of the drug}}$
pH	The inverse log of the hydrogen ion concentration	$pH = pK_a + \log \dfrac{\text{(unprotonated form)}}{\text{(protonated form)}}$
Half-life	The length of time required for 50% of a drug to be cleared from the system. (The equation applies to drugs eliminated by first-order kinetics.)	$t_{1/2} = \dfrac{0.693 \times V_d}{CL}$
Renal dose	The adjusted dose of a drug administered to patients with decreased renal function; takes into account the patient's renal function via creatinine clearance.	$\text{Corrected dose} = \text{average dose} \times \dfrac{\text{patient's creatinine clearance}}{100 \text{ mL / min}}$

DOSING

Type of Dose	Description	Equation
Maintenance Dose	The regimen used to achieve plasma concentration of a drug within the therapeutic window; a steady state, this value is equal to the elimination rate.	$\text{Dosing rate} = \dfrac{\text{clearance} \times \text{desired plasma concentration}}{\text{bioavailability}}$
Loading Dose	The dose required to achieve therapeutic plasma concentrations quickly.	$\text{Loading dose} = \dfrac{\text{Volume of distribution} \times \text{desired plasma concentration}}{\text{bioavailability}}$

THERAPEUTIC VALUES

Therapeutic Index (TI_{50})	• Numerical indication of the safety of a drug • The higher the value, the safer the drug • $TI_{50} = LD_{50} / ED_{50}$ • LD_{50}: the dose that is lethal in 50% of the population • ED_{50}: the dose that is effective in 50% of the population
Therapeutic Window	• The area between the minimum therapeutic concentration (trough) and the minimum concentration to produce toxicity (peak). • For some drugs, these values vary greatly from patient to patient and must be titrated for each patient. • For drugs with small therapeutic windows, smaller doses with more frequent dosing are preferred.

CHAPTER 2
ANTIMICROBIAL MEDICATIONS

VI. ANTIFUNGAL AGENTS

Mechanisms of Action and Classification of Antifungal Agents

Fungal Infections According to Commoness

Antifungals: Drug Facts

VII. ANTIPROTOZOAL AGENTS

Therapeutic Classification of Antiprotozoal Agents

Therapeutic Applications of Antiprotozoal Drugs

Antiprotozoals: Drug Facts

VIII. ANTIHELMINTHIC AGENTS

Antihelminthics: Drug Facts

IX. ANTIMYCOBACTERIAL AGENTS

Available agents for tuberculosis and leprosy plus atypical mycobacterial agents

Antimycobacterials: Drug Facts

Blackwater Fever	Syndrome of hemolytic anemia, hemoglobinuria, and renal failure associated with massive parasitemia.
Cinchonism	Poisoning syndrome associated with quinine, quinidine, and *Cinchona*; symptoms include tinnitus, deafness, headache, blurry vision, and nausea.
Disulfiram Reaction	Syndrome that occurs due to coingestion of alcohol and disulfiram; disulfiram blocks aldehyde dehydrogenase, leading to accumulation of acetaldehyde; symptoms include nausea, headache, flushing, and hypotension.
G6PD Deficiency	Lack of enzyme important in the oxidation/reduction capabilities of the red blood cell; deficiency leads to hydrogen peroxide accumulation, which causes hemolysis. Hemolysis often associated with drugs that produce oxidative stress (eg, sulfonamides).
Gray Baby Syndrome	Caused by deficiency of a hepatic enzyme required for the degradation of chloramphenicol; syndrome is characterized by circulatory collapse, cyanosis (gray color), and flaccidity in neonates.
Lassa Fever	A hemorrhage febrile illness associated with arenavirus infection.
Methemoglobinemia	Accumulation of methemoglobin, which is a form of hemoglobin with a low oxygen affinity. Methemoglobinemia results in pseudocyanosis, tissue hypoxia, and death.
Pseudomembranous Colitis	Inflammation of the colon caused by a toxin most often associated with *Clostridium difficile*; characterized by exudative plaques, also known as pseudomembranes; associated with antibiotic use such as clindamycin and ampicillin.
Stevens-Johnson Syndrome	Immunologic reaction characterized by lesions of the skin and mucous membranes; involves both the mouth and eyes.
Superinfection	A novel infection in addition to a preexisting one.
Trachoma	Chronic inflammation of the conjunctiva caused by *Chlamydia trachomatis*.

I. Cell Wall Synthesis Inhibitors

ANTIBIOTIC MECHANISMS OF ACTION

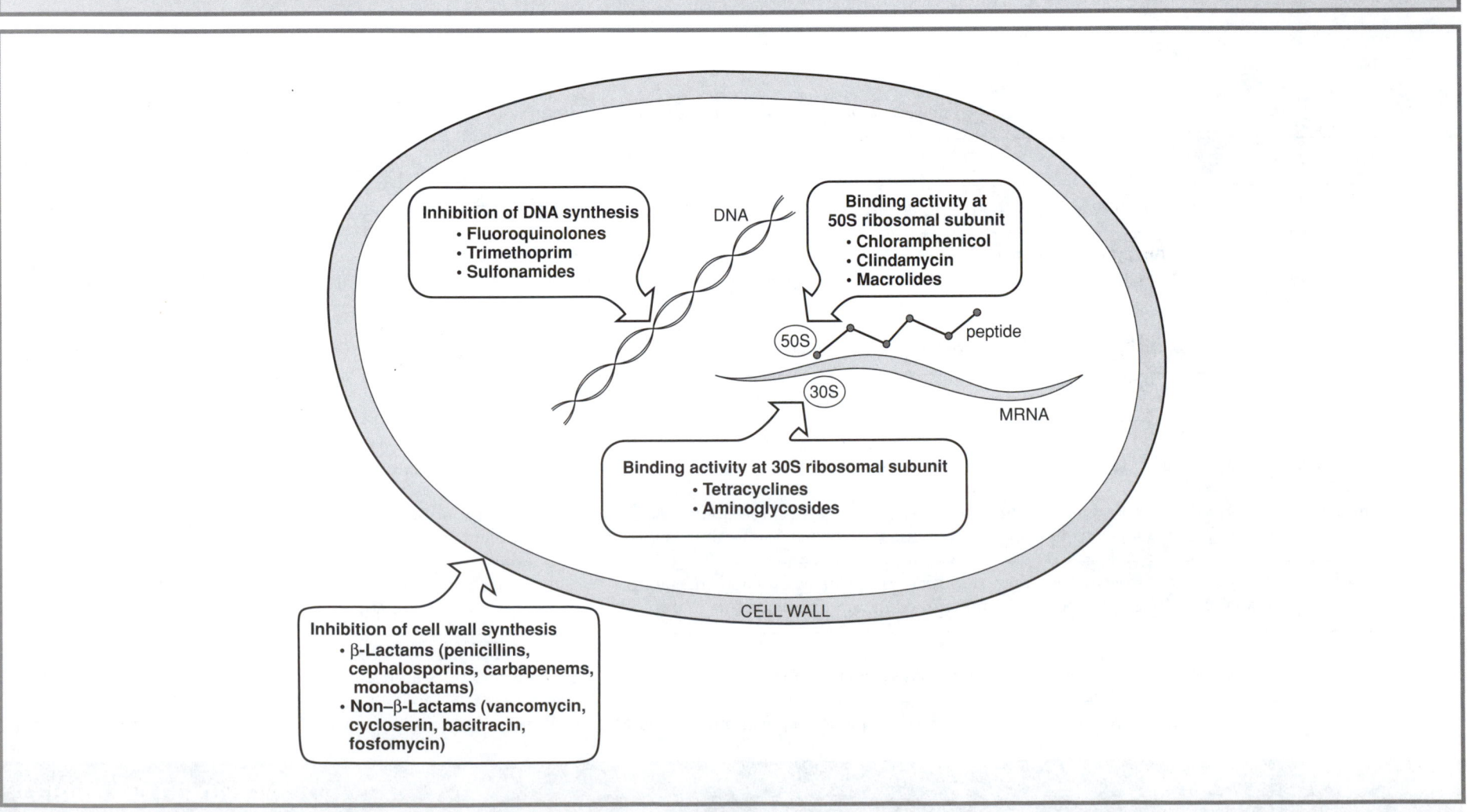

SUMMARY OF PENICILLINS

Types	Class	Pharmacokinetics	Mechanisms of Action and of Resistance	Clinical Uses and Spectrum of Activity	Drawbacks and Side Effects
Penicillin G and penicillin V	• Derivatives of 6-aminopenicillanic acid • Contain a β-lactam ring	• **A:** PO absorption inhibited by coingestion with meals • **M:** Polar compounds, so not extensively metabolized • **E:** Most are excreted in urine via glomerular filtration and tubular secretion; prolong effects by administration with Probenecid, which blocks tubular secretion	**MOA:** • Bactericidal • Inhibit cell wall synthesis by these three steps: 1. Bind drug to specific receptors in the bacterial cell wall 2. Inhibit transpeptidase enzymes that cross-link linear peptidoglycan chains that form bacterial cell walls 3. Activate autolytic enzymes causing lesions in the bacterial cell wall	• Narrow spectrum • β-Lactamase susceptible • Streptococci, meningococci, G+ bacilli, spirochetes	• Most staphylococci are drug resistant **Allergic reactions:** • Ranges from urticaria to hemolytic anemia and anaphylaxis • Assume cross-reactivity throughout class • 10% of persons who are allergic to penicillin are also allergic to cephalosporins
Methicillin, nafcillin, oxacillin, cloxacillin, and dicloxacillin				• Very narrow spectrum • β-Lactamase resistant • β-Lactamase–producing staphylococci	
Ampicillin and amoxicillin				• Wider spectrum • β-Lactamase susceptible • Similar therapeutic spectrum to narrow spectrum penicillins; also covers enterococci, *Listeria monocytogenes*, and *Moraxella catarrhalis* • Action enhanced when combined with inhibitors of β-lactamase (ie, clavulanic acid and sulbactam)	**GI disturbances:** • Nausea and diarrhea caused by oral medications via direct irritation or overgrowth of G+ organisms or yeast • Ampicillin implicated in pseudomembranous colitis **Cation toxicity:** • Possible toxic effects of Na+ or K+ when high doses of penicillin salts are used in patients with CV or renal disease
			Resistance: • β-Lactamase produced by bacteria causes enzymatic hydrolysis of the β-lactam ring, which results in loss of antibacterial activity		
Carbenicillin, piperacillin, and ticarcillin				• β-Lactamase susceptible • Similar therapeutic spectrum to narrow spectrum penicillins; also covers several G− rods (*Pseudomonas*, *Enterobacter*, and some *Klebsiella* species) • Action enhanced when combined with inhibitors of β-lactamase (ie, clavulanic acid and sulbactam)	

CLASSIFICATION OF PENICILLINS

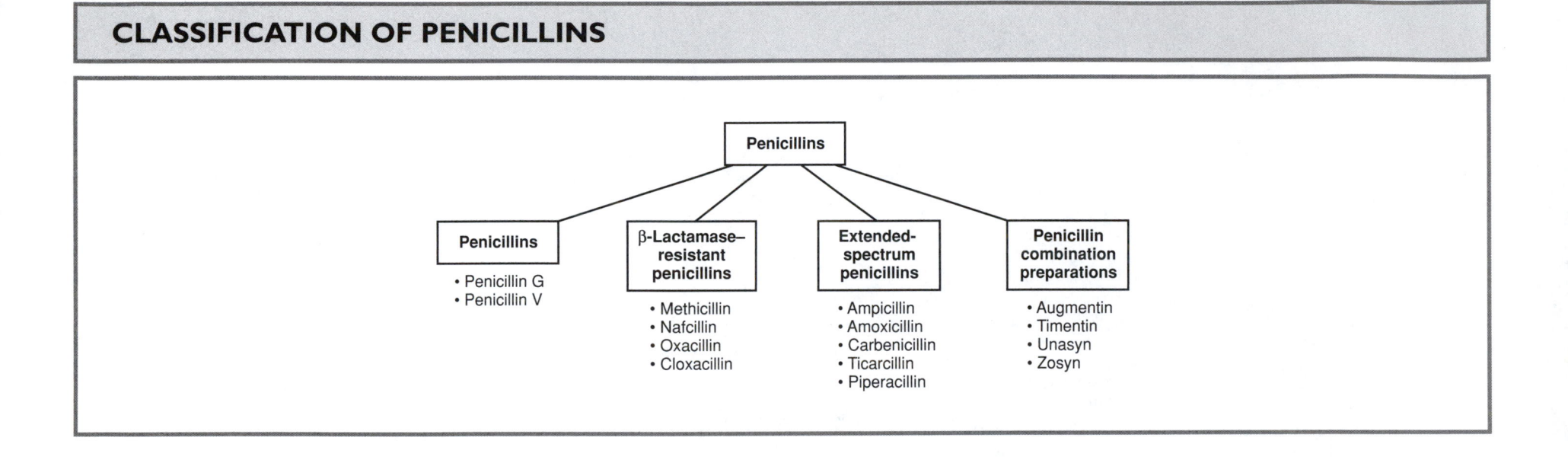

PENICILLINS AND β-LACTAMASE–RESISTANT PENICILLINS

Drug	Pharmacokinetics	Spectrum of Activity	Clinical Uses and General Information	Drawbacks and Side Effects
Penicillin G (Pentids, Pfizerpen)	• **A:** PO, IM or IV; 20% absorbed following PO administration (80% inactivated) • **B:** Low protein binding • **D:** Limited distribution; crosses BBB • **E:** Rapidly excreted unchanged in urine • Effects prolonged via IM administration of poorly soluble penicillin G salts, which dissolve slowly and enter the blood (ie, procaine penicillin G or benzathine penicillin G)	• G+ cocci (*Enterococcus, Staphylococcus, Streptococcus*) • G− cocci (*Neisseria*) • G+ bacilli (*Actinomyces, Bacillus, Clostridium, Corynebacterium, Listeria*) • Spirochetes (*Leptospira, Treponema*)	• Infections caused by bacteria listed in Spectrum of Activity column • First antibiotic discovered by Alexander Fleming in 1929	• Widespread resistance due to β-lactamase • Resistance develops quickly • Lack of PO administration • Broader spectrum preferable (lacks coverage of most G− organisms)
Penicillin V (Pen-Vee K, V-cillin)	• **A:** PO; absorbed in the duodenum (stable in acidic pH) • **B:** High protein binding • **D:** Widely distributed • **M:** Hepatic metabolism • **E:** Parent drug and metabolites excreted in urine		• Infections caused by bacteria listed in Spectrum of Activity column • Oropharyngeal infections	• Poor bioavailability • Narrow spectrum • Requires multiple daily dosing

Continued

PENICILLINS AND β-LACTAMASE–RESISTANT PENICILLINS (Continued)

Drug	Pharmacokinetics	Spectrum of Activity	Clinical Uses and General Information	Drawbacks and Side Effects
Methicillin (Staphcillin)	• **A:** IV and IM • **E:** Unchanged in urine	• β-Lactamase–producing *Staphylococcus* and *Streptococcus* ONLY • Not active against G− organisms	• Resistant staphylococcal infections • Nafcillin is more active against resistant strains than methicillin	• Can only be administered parenterally so it has limited uses • Nephrotoxicity • Neuropathy • Bone marrow depression • MRSA is treated with vancomycin
Nafcillin (Nallpen)	• **A:** IV, IM, and PO; erratic absorption with PO administration • **B:** High protein binding • **D:** Crosses the BBB • **E:** In feces			• Nephrotoxicity (less than methicillin) • Bone marrow depression
Oxacillin (Bactocill)	• **A:** IV and PO; well absorbed following PO administration • **M:** 60% metabolized to inactive metabolites by the liver; undergoes enterohepatic circulation • **E:** Metabolites excreted in urine			• Nephrotoxicity (less than methicillin) • Hepatotoxicity • Bone marrow depression
Cloxacillin (Tegopen)	• **A:** PO; well absorbed • **E:** Unchanged in urine			• Hepatotoxicity • Bone marrow depression

EXTENDED-SPECTRUM PENICILLINS

Drug	Pharmacokinetics	Spectrum of Activity	Clinical Uses and General Information	Drawbacks and Side Effects
Ampicillin (Ampicin)	• **A:** IV and PO; well absorbed with PO administration • **B:** Low protein binding • **D:** Widely distributed, crosses only inflamed meninges • **E:** Unchanged in urine	• G+ cocci (*Streptococcus, Enterococcus*) • G+ rods (*Clostridium, Listeria*) • G− cocci (*Neisseria*)	• UTI • Sinusitis • Otitis • Lower respiratory tract infections • Often used in combination with β-lactamase inhibitors	• β-Lactamase sensitive • Pseudomembranous colitis • Not useful for treating G+ infections (use penicillin G)
Amoxicillin (Amoxil, Trimox)	• **A:** PO; better absorbed than ampicillin following PO administration • **B:** Low protein binding • **D:** Widely distributed, only crosses inflamed meninges • **E:** Unchanged in urine	• G+ cocci (*Enterococcus, Staphylococcus, Streptococcus*) • G− cocci (*Neisseria*) • G− rods (*Escherichia coli, Haemophilus influenzae, Helicobacter pylori, Proteus*)	• ENT infections • GU infections • Lower respiratory tract infections • Skin infections	
Carbenicillin (Geocillin)	• **A:** PO; indanyl ester form for PO administration • **E:** Unchanged in urine	• G+ cocci (*Enterococcus*) • G− rods (*Enterobacter, E coli, Klebsiella, Morganella, Proteus, Pseudomonas*)	• UTIs • Prostatitis	• β-Lactamase sensitive • Often used in combination with β-lactamase inhibitors (see Combination Preparations of Penicillins chart) • Often combined with an aminoglycoside (cannot be mixed in same IV bag)

Continued

EXTENDED-SPECTRUM PENICILLINS (Continued)

Drug	Pharmacokinetics	Spectrum of Activity	Clinical Uses and General Information	Drawbacks and Side Effects
Ticarcillin (Ticar)	• **A:** IV • **B:** Low protein binding • **E:** Unchanged in urine	• G+ cocci (*Staphylococcus, Streptococcus, Enterococcus*) • G− cocci (*Neisseria*) • G− rods (non−β-lactamase producing forms of *Branhamella, Citrobacter, Enterobacter, E coli, H influenzae, Klebsiella, Morganella, Proteus, Providencia, Pseudomonas, Salmonella, Serratia*)	• GU infections • Intra-abdominal infections • Pneumonia • Septicemia • Skin infections	
Piperacillin (Pipracil)	• **A:** IV • **B:** Low plasma protein binding • **D:** Widely distributed; does not cross BBB • **E:** Unchanged in urine	• G+ cocci (*Streptococcus, Enterococcus*) • G+ bacilli (*Clostridium*) • G− cocci (*Neisseria*) • G− rods (*Bacteriodes, Citrobacter, Enterobacter, E coli, H influenzae, Klebsiella, Proteus, Pseudomonas, Serratia*)	• Bone and joint infections • Gynecologic infections • Intra-abdominal infections • Pneumonia • Septicemia • Skin infections • Surgical prophylaxis • UTIs	

COMBINATION PREPARATIONS OF PENICILLINS

Drug	Pharmacokinetics	Spectrum of Activity	Clinical Uses and General Information	Drawbacks and Side Effects
Amoxicillin and clavulinic acid (Augmentin)	• **A:** PO • See Amoxicillin	• G+ cocci (*Staphylococcus, Streptococcus, Enterococcus*) • G– cocci (*Neisseria*) • G– rods (*Bacteroides Eikenella, Enterobacter, E coli, Fusobacterium, H influenzae, Klebsiella, Moraxella, Proteus*)	• Bronchitis • Pneumonia • Otitis • Sinusitis • Skin infections • UTIs	• Clavulinic acid function to make it β-lactamase resistant
Ticarcillin and clavulinic acid (Timentin)	• **A:** IV • See Ticarcillin	• G+ cocci (*Staphylococcus, Streptococcus, Enterococcus*) • G+ bacilli (*Clostridium*) • G– cocci (*Neisseria*) • G– rods (*Bacteroides, Branhamella, Citrobacter, Enterobacter, E coli, Fusobacterium, H influenzae, Klebsiella, Morganella, Proteus, Providencia, Pseudomonas, Salmonella, Serratia*)	• Gynecologic infections • Intra-abdominal infections • Pneumonia • Septicemia • Skin infections • UTIs	• Local reactions at injection site • Tazobactam, sulbactam, and clavulinic acid function to make these β-lactamase resistant
Ampicillin and Sulbactam (Unasyn)	• **A:** IV or IM • See Ampicillin	• G+ cocci (*Staphylococcus, Streptococcus, Enterococcus*) • G+ rods (*Clostridium*) • G– cocci (*Neisseria*) • G– rods (*Bacteroides, E coli, H influenzae, Klebsiella, Moraxella, Proteus, Providencia*)	• Gynecologic infections • Intra-abdominal infections • Skin infections	
Piperacillin and Tazobactam (Zosyn)	• **A:** IV • See Piperacillin	• G+ cocci (*Staphylococcus, Streptococcus, Enterococcus*) • G+ rods (*Clostridium*) • G– cocci (*Neisseria*) • G– rods (*Bacteroides, Fusobacterium, Klebsiella, Moraxella, Morganella, Proteus, Pseudomonas, Serratia*)	• Gynecologic infections • Intra-abdominal infections • Pneumonia • Skin infections	

CLASSIFICATION OF CEPHALOSPORINS

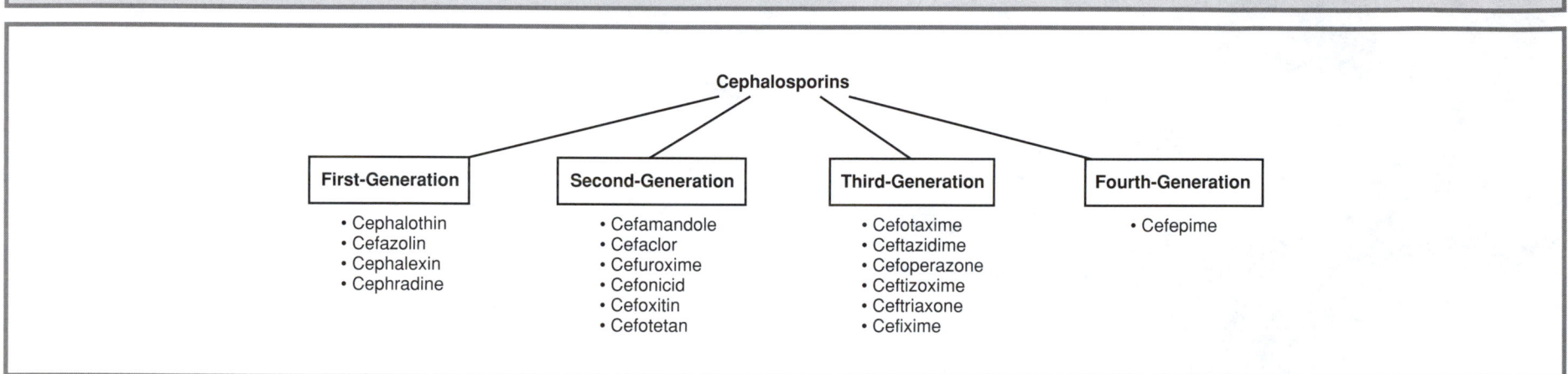

Cephalosporins

First-Generation
- Cephalothin
- Cefazolin
- Cephalexin
- Cephradine

Second-Generation
- Cefamandole
- Cefaclor
- Cefuroxime
- Cefonicid
- Cefoxitin
- Cefotetan

Third-Generation
- Cefotaxime
- Ceftazidime
- Cefoperazone
- Ceftizoxime
- Ceftriaxone
- Cefixime

Fourth-Generation
- Cefepime

SUMMARY OF CEPHALOSPORINS

Type*	Pharmacokinetics	Mechanisms of Action and of Resistance	Spectrum of Activity	Clinical Uses and General Information	Drawbacks and Side Effects
First-generation	• **A:** IV and PO • **D:** Most first- and second-generation cephalosporins do not cross BBB, even with inflamed meninges • **M:** Cephalosporins with side chains may undergo hepatic metabolism • **E:** Majority excreted unchanged in urine via active tubular secretion; EXCEPT cefoperazone and ceftriaxone, which are mainly excreted in bile	**MOA:** • Bactericidal • Bind to site on organism cell wall • Inhibit cell wall synthesis **Resistance:** • Less resistance than seen with penicillins because cephalosporins have a more stable β-lactam ring • Via production of β-lactamase • Via decreased membrane permeability to cephalosporins • Via mutation in the binding site on cell membrane	• Best for G+ cocci • Susceptible to β-lactamase	• Surgical prophylaxis	**Allergic reactions:** 5–15% of persons allergic to penicillin are also allergic to cephalosporins • Anaphylaxis (contraindicated in patients with penicillin anaphylaxis) • Fever • Skin rash • Nephritis • Granulocytopenia • Hemolytic anemia **Other reactions:** • MTT side chain: causes hypoprothrombinemia and inhibits aldehyde dehydrogenase (can cause disulfiram-like reaction with alcohol ingestion) • Local irritation (at injection site) and thrombophlebitis • Increase nephrotoxicity of aminoglycosides when administered together
Second-generation			• Extended G− coverage • Less activity against G+ organisms than first generation	• Parenteral administration required (except for cefaclor)	
Third-generation			• Exquisitely active against G− bacilli • Not useful for G+ infections	• All administered parenterally (except for cefixime) • Almost all cross BBB • Generally reserved for serious infections (ie, bacterial meningitis)	
Fourth-generation			• G+ activity of first-generation • Best for G− organisms • More resistant to β-lactamases produced by G− organisms	• Better for infections caused by β-lactamase–producing G− organisms including *Enterobacter*, *Haemophilus*, *Neisseria* • In general, to prevent resistance, administer cephalosporins with other agents such as aminoglycosides. • Generally, cephalosporins are used prophylactically • As the generation increases, so does the potency and spectrum, especially against G− species (decreases somewhat against G+ species)	

*All contain the β-lactam ring.

EFFECTIVENESS OF CEPHALOSPORINS AGAINST G− AND G+ ORGANISMS

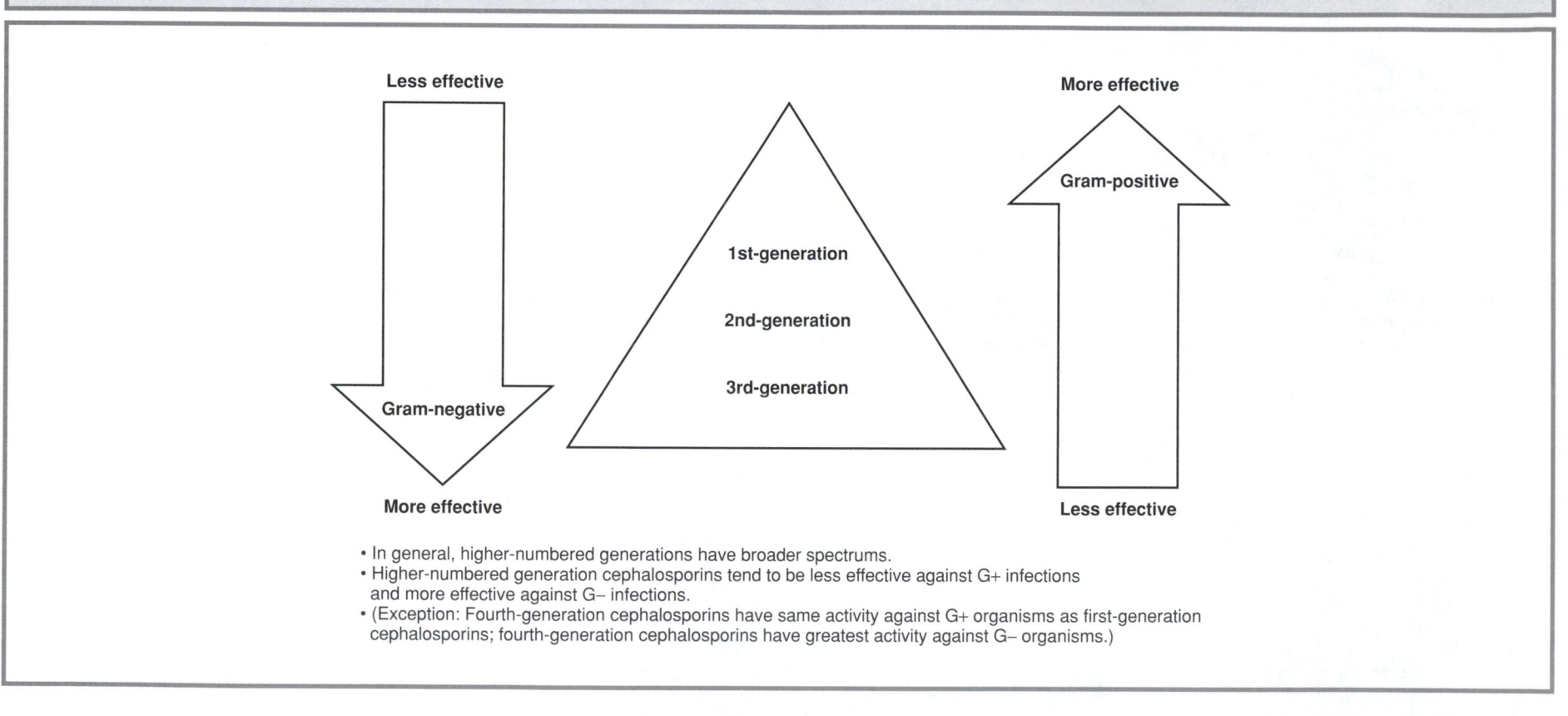

- In general, higher-numbered generations have broader spectrums.
- Higher-numbered generation cephalosporins tend to be less effective against G+ infections and more effective against G− infections.
- (Exception: Fourth-generation cephalosporins have same activity against G+ organisms as first-generation cephalosporins; fourth-generation cephalosporins have greatest activity against G− organisms.)

FIRST-GENERATION CEPHALOSPORINS

Drug	Pharmacokinetics	Spectrum of Activity	Clinical Uses and General Information	Drawbacks and Side Effects
Cephalothin (Keflin)	• **A:** IM (associated with pain at site); IV (associated with thrombophlebitis so no longer used) • $t_{1/2}$: 30–60 minutes • **E:** In urine	• Best generation cephalosporins for G+ infections • Susceptible to β-lactamases	• Surgical prophylaxis • Pneumonia • UTI	**Allergic reactions:** 5–15% of persons allergic to penicillin are also allergic to cephalosporins • Anaphylaxis (contraindicated in patients with penicillin anaphylaxis) • Fever
Cefazolin (Ancef, Kefzol)	• **A:** IV and IM • **D:** Penetrates well into most tissues; does not cross BBB • $t_{1/2}$: 1.4–2 hours • **E:** Unchanged in urine		• Surgical prophylaxis • Pneumonia • UTI	• Skin rash • Nephritis • Granulocytopenia • Hemolytic anemia **Other reactions:**
Cephalexin (Keflex)	• **A:** PO • $t_{1/2}$: 0.9–1.5 hours • **E:** Unchanged in urine		• Pharyngitis • Tonsillitis • Skin and soft tissue infections	• Local irritation (at injection site) and thrombophlebitis • Increase nephrotoxicity of aminoglycosides when administered together
Cephradine (Anspor, Velosef)	• **A:** PO, IV, and IM • $t_{1/2}$: 1.3 hours • **E:** Unchanged in urine		• UTI • Skin and soft tissue infections • Pneumonia • Prostatitis	

SECOND-GENERATION CEPHALOSPORINS

Drug	Pharmacokinetics	Spectrum of Activity	Clinical Uses and General Information	Drawbacks and Side Effects
Cefamandole (Mandol)	• **A:** IV and IM • $t_{1/2}$: 0.5–1.2 hours • **E:** Unchanged in urine	• More G— coverage than first-generation cephalosporins • Less G+ coverage than first-generation cephalosporins	• Surgical prophylaxis • Skin and soft tissue infections • Pneumonia	**Allergic reactions:** 5–15% of persons allergic to penicillin are also allergic to cephalosporins • Anaphylaxis (contraindicated in patients with penicillin anaphylaxis) • Fever • Skin rash • Nephritis • Granulocytopenia • Hemolytic anemia
Cefaclor (Ceclor)	• **A:** PO • $t_{1/2}$: 0.6–0.9 hours • **E:** Unchanged in urine		• Pharyngitis • Tonsillitis • Otitis • Pneumonia • UTI • Skin and soft tissue infections	
Cefuroxime (Ceftin, Kefurox)	• **A:** PO and IM • **D:** Only second-generation drug to cross BBB • $t_{1/2}$: 1.2–1.9 hours • **E:** Unchanged in urine		• Pharyngitis • Tonsillitis • UTI • Skin and soft tissue infections • Bronchitis • Gonorrhea • Lyme disease	**Other reactions:** • MTT side chain: causes hypo-prothrombinemia and inhibits aldehyde dehydrogenase (can cause disulfiram-like reaction with alcohol ingestion); seen with cefamandole and cefotetan • Local irritation (at injection site) and thrombophlebitis • Increase nephrotoxicity of aminoglycosides when administered together
Cefonicid (Monocid)	• **A:** IV and IM • $t_{1/2}$: 3.5–4.5 hours • **E:** Unchanged in urine		• Surgical prophylaxis • UTI	

Cefoxitin (Mefoxin)	• **A:** IM and IV • $t_{1/2}$: 0.7–1.1 hours • **E:** Majority excreted unchanged in urine	• Surgical prophylaxis (especially for abdominal surgery and for mixed anaerobic infections such as those found in peritonitis and diverticulitis)
Cefotetan (Cefotan)	• **A:** IM and IV • $t_{1/2}$: 3–4.6 hours • **E:** Unchanged in urine	• Surgical prophylaxis • UTI • Skin and soft tissue infections

THIRD- AND FOURTH-GENERATION CEPHALOSPORINS

Drug	Pharmacokinetics	Spectrum of Activity	Clinical Uses and General Information	Drawbacks and Side Effects
Cefotaxime (Claforan)	• **A:** IM and IV • **D:** Widely distributed; crosses BBB • $t_{1/2}$: 1 hour • **E:** Parent drug and metabolites excreted in urine	• Exquisitely active against G— bacilli • Not useful for G+ infections	• Surgical prophylaxis • Septicemia • Gonorrhea	**Allergic reactions:** 5–15% of persons allergic to penicillin are also allergic to cephalosporins • Anaphylaxis (contraindicated in patients with penicillin anaphylaxis) • Fever
Ceftazidime (Ceptaz, Fortaz)	• **A:** IM and IV • **D:** Widely distributed; crosses BBB • $t_{1/2}$: 1.4–2 hours • **E:** Unchanged in urine		• UTIs • Pneumonia • Bone and joint infections • Intra-abdominal infections • Septicemia • Skin and soft tissue infections	• Skin rash • Nephritis • Granulocytopenia • Hemolytic anemia **Other reactions:**
Cefoperazone (Cefobid)	• **A:** IM and IV • **D:** Widely distributed; does not cross BBB • $t_{1/2}$: 1.6–2.4 hours • **E:** Majority excreted unchanged in feces; remainder unchanged in urine		• Severe infections (including pyelonephritis)	• MTT side chain: causes hypoprothrombinemia and inhibits aldehyde dehydrogenase (can cause disulfiram-like reaction with alcohol ingestion); seen with cefoperazone • Local irritation (at injection site) and thrombophlebitis • Increase nephrotoxicity of aminoglycosides when administered together
Ceftizoxime (Cefizox)	• **A:** IM and IV • $t_{1/2}$: 1.4–1.7 hours • **E:** Unchanged in urine		• PID • UTI • Gonorrhea	

Ceftriaxone (Rocephin)	• **A:** IM and IV • $t_{1/2}$: 4.3–8.7 hours • **E:** Unchanged in feces and urine		• Meningitis • Skin and soft tissue infections • Surgical prophylaxis • Gonorrhea
Cefixime (Suprax)	• **A:** PO • $t_{1/2}$: 3–4 hours • **E:** Majority excreted unchanged in urine		• Bronchitis • Pharyngitis • Tonsillitis • UTI • Gonorrhea
Cefepime (Maxipime)*	• **A:** IM and IV • **D:** Widely distributed; crosses BBB • $t_{1/2}$: 2 hours • **E:** Majority excreted unchanged in urine	• Same activity against G+ organisms as first-generation cephalosporins • Greatest activity against G– organisms • Good activity against *Pseudomonas*, Enterobacteriaceae, *Staphylococcus aureus*, and *Streptococcus pneumoniae*	• Intra-abdominal infections • Skin and soft tissue infections • UTI • Pneumonia • Neutropenic fever

*Indicates only fourth-generation cephalosporin in the table.

OTHER β-LACTAMS

Drug	Pharmacokinetics	Spectrum of Activity	Clinical Uses and General Information	Drawbacks and Side Effects
Carbapenem				
Imipenem (Primaxin)	• **A:** IM and IV • **D:** Penetrates tissues well; crosses BBB • **M:** Inactivated in renal tubules (coadministered with cilastatin, which inhibits this enzymatic inactivation) • **E:** In urine	• G− rods • G+ organisms • Anaerobes	• Reserved for infections resistant to other medications • Less susceptible to β-lactamase inactivation	• GI distress • Skin rash • CNS toxicity (ie, seizures, confusion)
Meropenem (Merrem)	• **A:** IV • **D:** Penetrates tissues well; crosses BBB • **E:** Unchanged in urine	• Similar spectrum to imipenem • Greater activity against G− aerobes • Less effective against G+ organisms	• Reserved for infections resistant to other medications • Less susceptible to β-lactamase inactivation • Not metabolized by renal tubule enzymes therefore does not require cilastatin coadministration • Less risk of CNS toxicity than imipenem	• GI distress • Skin rash
Monobactam				
Aztreonam (Azactam)	• **A:** IM and IV • **E:** Majority excreted unchanged in urine	• G− rods	• Clinical use not well defined • Relatively resistant to β-lactamase inactivation • Can be used in patients who are allergic to penicillin	• Skin rashes • Elevation of serum aminotransferases

OTHER CELL WALL SYNTHESIS INHIBITORS: NON–β-LACTAMS

Drug	Pharmacokinetics	Mechanisms of Action and of Resistance	Spectrum	Clinical Uses	Drawbacks and Side Effects
Vancomycin (Vancocin)	• **A:** IV and PO; PO form poorly absorbed so only used for colitis caused by *Clostridium difficile* • **D:** Widely distributed; crosses inflamed meninges • **E:** 90% excreted unchanged in urine	**MOA:** • Binds to end of nascent protein • This inhibits transglycosylase, which elongates the protein • Thus, elongation and cross-linking are prevented **Resistance:** • Via modification at binding site on peptidoglycan	• G+ organisms	• Used for serious infections caused by drug-resistant G+ organisms • Infections caused by MRSA • Infections caused by penicillin-resistant pneumococci • Infections caused by *C difficile*	• Chills • Fever • Phlebitis • Ototoxicity • Nephrotoxicity
Cycloserine (Seromycin, Pulvules)	• **A:** PO • **D:** Widely distributed • **E:** Majority excreted unchanged in urine	**MOA:** • Structural analog of D-alanine • Inhibits incorporation of D-alanine into pentapeptide side chain of peptidoglycan	• G+ organisms • G− organisms	• Infections caused by *Mycobacterium tuberculosis* that is resistant to other first-line agents	• CNS toxicity (eg, headaches, tremors, psychosis)
Bacitracin (Baciguent, Neosporin)	• **A:** Topical • **E:** Small absorbed amounts are excreted in urine	**MOA:** • Interferes with late stage of cell wall synthesis	• G+ organisms	• Suppression of flora in surface abrasions or wounds	• Nephrotoxic (so only used topically)
Fosfomycin (Monurol)	• **A:** PO and IV (only PO approved in United States) • **E:** Unchanged in urine	**MOA:** • Interferes with early stage of cell wall synthesis **Resistance:** • Via inadequate transport of the drug into the cell	• G+ organisms • G− organisms	• Uncomplicated UTIs	• Diarrhea

II. 30S Antibacterial Agents

AMINOGLYCOSIDES

Drug	Pharmacokinetics		Mechanisms of Action and of Resistance	Spectrum of Activity	Clinical Uses and General Information	Drawbacks and Side Effects
Streptomycin	• **A:** IM	• **A:** PO, poor absorption due to ionization; IM and IV, good absorption • **D:** Widely distributed, enters CNS only with inflamed meninges • **E:** In urine	**MOA:** • Bactericidal • Binds to 30S ribosomal subunit • Causes abnormal peptide synthesis • Synergistic action with β-lactams **Resistance:** • Via genetic change leading to impaired drug entry into the cell • Via mutation at the binding site on the 30S ribosomal subunit • Via enzymatic degradation by organism	• Aerobic G— rods (uptake of drug is an oxygen-dependent process) • Limited activity against facultative anaerobes in the presence of oxygen	• Tuberculosis (second-line agent) • Bubonic plague • Tularemia • *Pseudomonas* • Streptococcal endocarditis	• Drug resistance is fairly widespread (therefore they are often used with second- and third-generation cephalosporins) • Optic nerve toxicity (seen with streptomycin)
Neomycin (Mycifradin)	• **A:** PO				• Only used topically (most nephrotoxic so not used systemically) • Skin infections • Bowel sterilization	• Allergic skin reactions (most seen with neomycin) • Neuromuscular blockade—rare (decreased Ach release at NMJ can cause respiratory paralysis)
Gentamicin (Garamycin, Jenamicin)	• **A:** IM, IV				• Most frequently used • Tobramycin is less nephrotoxic	• Cannot be physically mixed with β-lactams due to acid/base neutralization reaction • Nephrotoxicity (proximal tubular cells) • Ototoxicity (acoutic portion), also occurs in unborn fetus
Tobramycin (Nebcin)						

| Amikacin (Amikin) | | • Used to treat streptomycin-resistant M *tuberculosis*

 • Effective against many organisms resistant to tobramycin and gentamicin |  **AMINO**

 A–**A**llergic skin reactions
 M–neuro**M**uscular blockade
 I–**I**nactivated when physically mixed with β-lactams
 N–**N**ephrotoxic
 O–**O**totoxic, **O**ptic nerve toxicity |
| Netilmicin (Netrimycin) | | • Reserved as a backup drug for organisms resistant to other aminoglycosides

 • Less toxic

 • Less susceptible to bacterial inactivation | |

TETRACYCLINES

Drug	Pharmacokinetics	Mechanisms of Action and of Resistance	Spectrum of Activity	Clinical Uses	Drawbacks and Side Effects
Tetracycline (Achromycin V)	• **A:** PO, topical	**MOA:**	• G+ organisms	• Drugs of choice for	• Bony structure dysplasia and discoloration; also occurs in fetus
	• **A:** PO, decent GI absorption (impaired when taken with foods containing calcium, iron, or aluminum); IV, can inhibit platelet aggregation; IM or SC, painful	• Bacteriostatic	• G− organisms	– *Vibrio cholerae*	
Oxytetracycline (Terramycin)	**A:** PO, IM	• Enter organism via diffusion or via active transport pump	• anaerobes	– *Acne*	• Photosensitivity
				– *Chlamydia*	
		• Bind (reversibly) to 30S ribosomal subunit		– *Ureaplasma urealyticum*	• GI irritation; eg, nausea, vomiting, and diarrhea
	• **D:** Extremely good distribution; crosses healthy meninges and placenta			– *Mycoplasma*	
Demeclocycline (Declomycin)	**A:** PO	• Slow protein synthesis		– Tularemia	• Alters normal flora; can precipitate pseudomembranous colitis caused by C *difficile*
		Resistance:		– *Borrelia burgdorferi*	
	• **E:** Enterohepatic cycling; glomerular filtration EXCEPT doxycycline, which undergoes hepatic inactivation and biliary excretion	• Via impaired transport pump (decreased influx or increased efflux)		– *Rickettsia*	
Minocycline (Minocin)	**A:** PO			☞ **VACUuM** The **B**ed**R**oom	• Hepatotoxicity, usually in pregnant women
		• Via mutation at the ribosomal subunit binding site		• Demeclocycline can treat SIADH by inhibiting the action of ADH at the renal tubule	• Nephrotoxicity
		• Via enzymatic inactivation			• Vestibular reactions; eg, vertigo, dizziness, nausea and vomiting
Doxycycline (Vibramycin)	**A:** PO, IV				

III. 50S Antibacterial Agents

MACROLIDES, CLINDAMYCIN, AND CHLORAMPHENICOL

Drug	Pharmacokinetics	Mechanisms of Action and of Resistance	Spectrum of Activity and Clinical Uses	Drawbacks and Side Effects
Erythromycin (E-Mycin)*	• **A:** PO; requires enteric coated tablets or acid-resistant salts since they are inactivated by acid; erythromycin also available in IV and topical forms • **D:** Distributes to most body compartments, only crosses inflamed meninges • **E:** Released into bile and feces as active drug (good for biliary infections)	**MOA:** • Bacteriostatic • Binds to the 50S subunit and blocks protein synthesis **Resistance:** • Develops mostly by mutations in the binding site on the 50S subunit	• G+ organisms • *Mycoplasma pneumoniae* • *Chlamydia* (good for pregnant women) • *Legionella pneumoniae* • *Campylobacter jejuni* • Active metabolite formed in liver acts synergistically with parent drug • Duration of action allows for 12-hour dosing • Decreases P450 activity	• Acts on cytochrome P450 system in liver and can cause drug interactions (eg, theophylline and carbamezepine) • GI upset • Abdominal cramping • Gas and diarrhea • Intestinal superinfection (very rare) • Cholestatic hepatitis with estolate salt form
Clarithromycin (Biaxin)*			• Same spectrum as erythromycin plus *H influenzae*, *Bordetella*, and *M catarrhalis* • Active metabolite formed in liver acts synergistically with parent drug • Duration of action allows for 12-hour dosing • Decreases P450 activity	

*Macrolides have large cyclic lactone ring structures with attached sugars.

Continued

MACROLIDES, CLINDAMYCIN, AND CHLORAMPHENICOL (Continued)

Drug	Pharmacokinetics	Mechanisms of Action and of Resistance	Spectrum of Activity and Clinical Uses	Drawbacks and Side Effects
Azithromycin (Zithromax)*	See page 37.	See page 37.	• Same erythromycin plus *H influenzae*, *Moraxella*, and *Chlamydia* • Taken up by phagocytes, transported to area of infection • 24-hour dosing; 5 day cycle	See page 37.
Clindamycin (Cleocin, Dalacin)	• **A:** PO, IV, IM, and topical; good tissue penetration after oral absorption	**MOA:** • Inhibit bacterial protein synthesis similarly to macrolides **Resistance:** • Via methylation of the binding site on the 50S ribosomal subunit • Via enzymatic inactivation	• G+ cocci and *B fragilis* • Prophylaxis in orthopedic surgery and treatment of osteomyelitis because of its ability to concentrate in bones	• Use has led to the emergence of pseudomembranous colitis caused by *C difficile*
Chloramphenicol (Chloromycetin)	• **A:** PO (well absorbed), IV, IM • **D:** Penetrates all tissues well including healthy meninges • **E:** 90% is glucuronidated and excreted in the urine	**MOA:** • Bacteriostatic • Bactericidal for *H influenzae* • Inhibits activity of bacterial 50S ribosomal subunit **Resistance:** • Via enzymatic inactivation (does not occur in *Rickettsia* species)	• Very broad spectrum of activity (G+ and G−) • First choice for *H influenzae* in children	• Bone marrow suppression that can be reversible or irreversible • Hypersensitivity reaction (unpredictable) • Toxic to neonates • Gray baby syndrome

*Macrolides have large cyclic lactone ring structures with attached sugars.

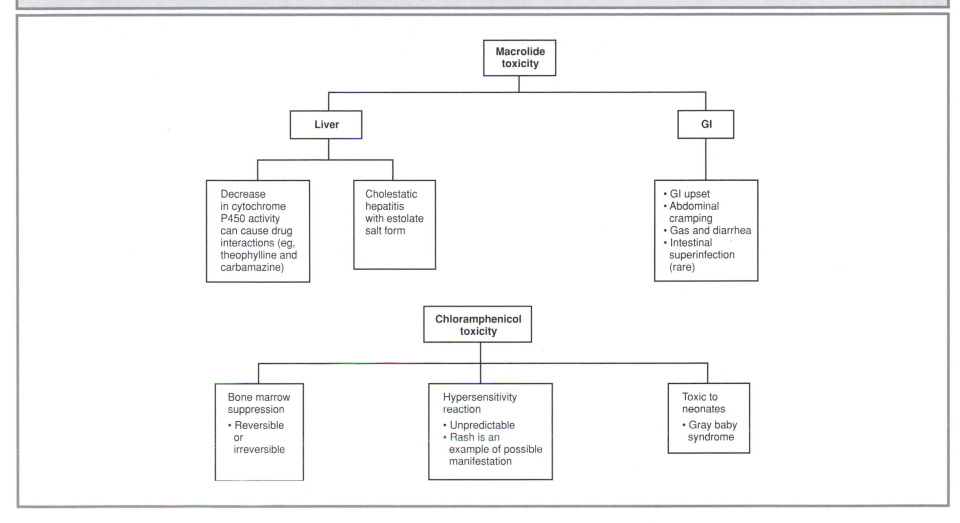

IV. Other Antibacterial Agents

CLASSIFICATION OF OTHER ANTIBACTERIAL AGENTS

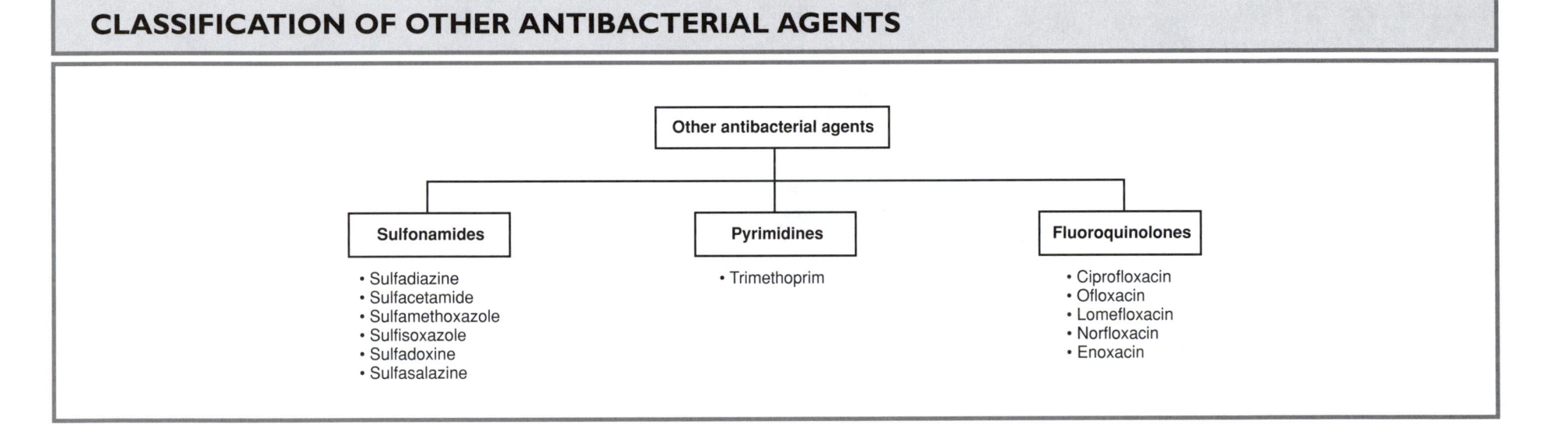

SULFONAMIDES, TRIMETHOPRIM, AND FLUOROQUINOLONES

Drugs	Pharmacokinetics		Mechanisms of Action and of Resistance	Spectrum of Activity	Clinical Uses	Drawbacks and Side Effects
Sulfonamides						
Sulfadiazine (Coptin)	• **A:** Topical	• **A:** PO; absorbed from the stomach and small intestine	**MOA:** • Bacteriostatic • Structural analogs of PABA	• G+ organisms • G– organisms • *Chlamydia* • *Nocardia*	• Prevention of burn infections	• Widespread drug resistance **Local effects:**
Sulfacetamide (Sulamyd, Bleph-10)	• **A:** Topical	• **D:** Readily distributed to all tissues (including CSF and placenta)	• Competitively inhibit the conversion of PABA to folic acid by dihydropteroate synthase		• Ocular infections (eg, conjunctivitis and trachoma)	• Irritation • Stinging • Burning
Sulfamethoxazole/ SMZ (Gantanol)	• **A:** PO	• **M:** Acetylated or glucuronidated by the liver to inactive toxic metabolites	• Lack of folic acid inhibits bacterial growth by interfering with microbial DNA synthesis		• UTI • Respiratory tract infections • Otitis media • Pneumonia • Dysentery	**Systemic effects:** • Fever • Rashes • Photosensitivity • Vomiting
Sulfisoxazole (Gantrisin pediatric)	• **A:** PO	• **E:** Active drug and inactive metabolites excreted into urine by glomerular filtration	**Resistance:** • Via microbial overproduction of PABA • Via loss of cell permeability to sulfonamides • Via structural changes that occur in bacterial dihydropteroate synthase		Sulfisoxazole plus phenazopyridine (a urinary analgesic) for UTI • Respiratory tract infections • Otitis media • Pneumonia • Dysentery	• Diarrhea • Stevens-Johnson syndrome • Rare hematopoietic disturbances • Can precipitate in neutral or acidic urine causing crystalluria, hematuria, or obstruction

Continued

Drugs	Pharmacokinetics	Mechanisms of Action and of Resistance	Spectrum of Activity	Clinical Uses	Drawbacks and Side Effects
Sulfadoxine	• **A:** PO See page 41.	See page 41.	See page 41.	• Sulfadoxine plus pyrimethamine is a second-line agent for malaria prophylaxis • Sulfadoxine plus quinine as first-line treatment of malaria	See page 41.
Sulfasalazine (Azulfidine)	• **A:** PO			• Enterocolitis and other IBD • Ulcerative colitis	
Pyrimidines					
Trimethoprim/ TMP	• **A:** PO and IV; well absorbed from GI tract • **D:** Readily distributed to most tissues (including CSF) • **E:** Most is excreted in unchanged urine, some is biotransformed into inactive products	**MOA:** • Bacteriostatic (almost bactericidal when combined with sulfonamides) • Inhibits dihydrofolate reductase • Inhibits bacterial growth by interfering with microbial DNA synthesis • Synergistic with sulfonamides **Resistance:** • Via reduced cell permeability • Via overproduction of dihydrofolate reductase • Via microbial modification of enzyme with decreased drug binding	• G+ organisms • G− organisms	**Alone:** • Acute UTIs **With Sulfamethoxazole:** • PCP • Shigellosis • GI infections • Systemic *Salmonella* infections • UTIs • Respiratory infections caused by *H influenzae*, *Moraxella*, *Klebsiella*, or *S pneumoniae* • Prophylaxis for PCP in immunosuppressed patients • G− sepsis	• Nausea, vomiting, and diarrhea • Drug fever • CNS disturbances • Rashes • Rare hematopoietic disturbances

Fluoroquinolones

Ciprofloxacin (Cipro)	• **A:** Topical, PO, IV	• **A:** Well absorbed PO • **D:** Widely distributed to most tissues • **M:** Some are biotransformed by liver to inactive metabolites • **E:** Most are eliminated either by tubular secretion or glomerular filtration	**MOA:** • Bactericidal • Prevents DNA unwinding required for transcription and translation by inhibiting DNA gyrase **Resistance:** • Via alteration of membrane permeability into the bacterial cell • Via microbial modification of DNA gyrase structure	• G+ organisms • G− organisms • *Chlamydia*	• Conjunctivitis, corneal ulcer, and other superficial ocular infections • Drug resistant UTIs • Lower respiratory tract infections • Bone, joint, skin, and skin structure infections • Infectious diarrhea • Typhoid fever • Gonococcal infections
Ofloxacin (Floxin)	• **A:** Topical, PO, IV				
Lomefloxacin (Maxaquim)	• **A:** PO				
Norfloxacin (Noroxin)	• **A:** PO; least well absorbed of the fluoro-quinolones				
Enoxacin (Penetrex)	• **A:** PO				

Additional column (adverse effects):
• Contraindicated in patients younger than 18 years because of the possibility of damage to growing cartilage
• Nausea
• Diarrhea
• Skin rashes
• Abnormal LFTs
• Very rarely CNS effects like headache and tremor
• Risk of tendonitis and tendon rupture

ANTIBACTERIAL SYNERGY OF SULFONAMIDES AND TRIMETHOPRIM

Inhibition of two successive steps in tetrahydrofolic acid formation results in antibacterial synergy.

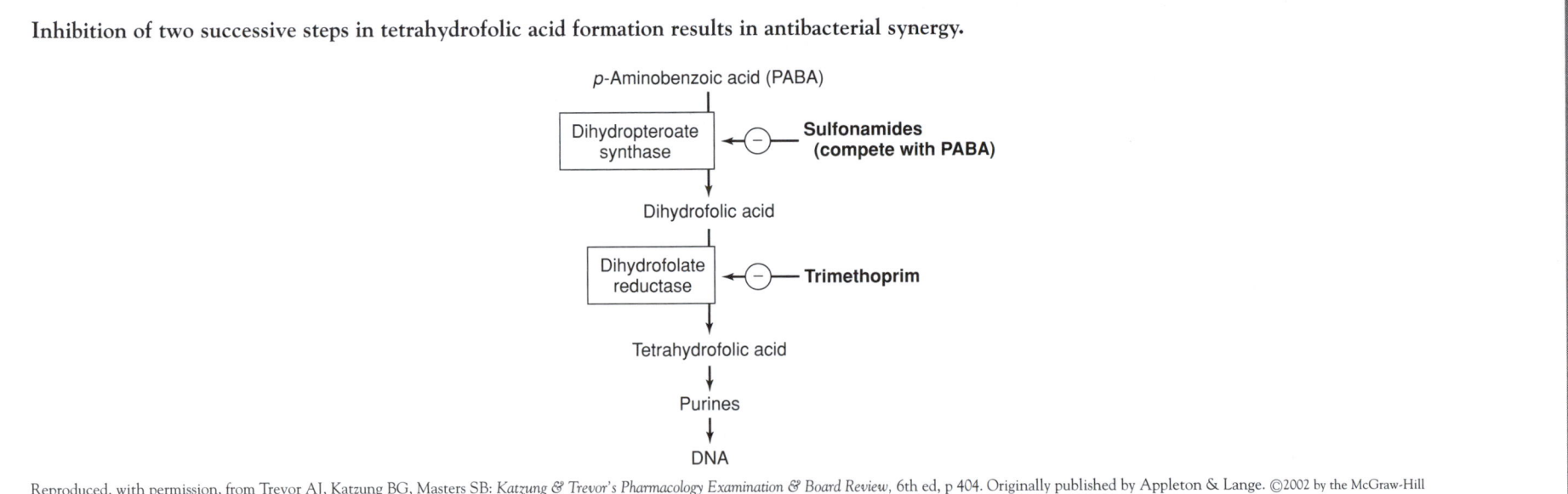

Reproduced, with permission, from Trevor AJ, Katzung BG, Masters SB: *Katzung & Trevor's Pharmacology Examination & Board Review*, 6th ed, p 404. Originally published by Appleton & Lange. ©2002 by the McGraw-Hill Companies, Inc.

V. Antiviral Agents

CLASSIFICATION OF ANTIVIRAL AGENTS

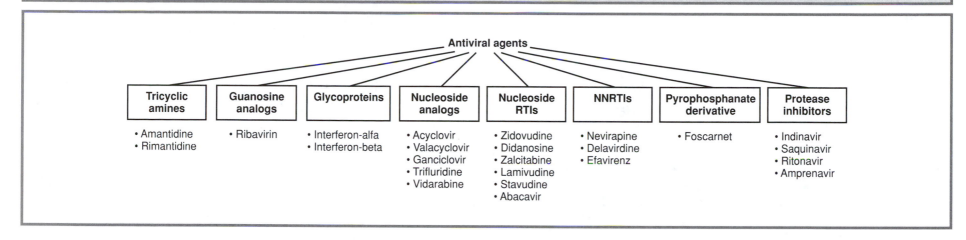

Antiviral agents

Tricyclic amines	Guanosine analogs	Glycoproteins	Nucleoside analogs	Nucleoside RTIs	NNRTIs	Pyrophosphanate derivative	Protease inhibitors
• Amantidine • Rimantidine	• Ribavirin	• Interferon-alfa • Interferon-beta	• Acyclovir • Valacyclovir • Ganciclovir • Trifluridine • Vidarabine	• Zidovudine • Didanosine • Zalcitabine • Lamivudine • Stavudine • Abacavir	• Nevirapine • Delavirdine • Efavirenz	• Foscarnet	• Indinavir • Saquinavir • Ritonavir • Amprenavir

TRICYLIC AMINES, GUANOSINE ANALOG, GLYCOPROTEINS, AND PYROPHOSPHONATE DERIVATIVE

Drug	Pharmacokinetics	Mechanisms of Action and of Resistance	Clinical Uses	Drawbacks and Side Effects
Tricyclic Amines				
Amantadine (Symmetrel)	• **A:** PO, rapidly absorbed from GI tract • **D:** Crosses BBB • **E:** Unchanged in urine	**MOA:** • Blocks viral RNA uncoating of influenza A, inhibiting viral replication • Causes dopamine release in CNS	• Prophylaxis for influenza A • Influenza treatment • Initial therapy for Parkinson's disease (due to DA release triggered in CNS)	• GI irritation • Dizziness • Ataxia • Slurred speech
Rimantadine (Flumadine)	• **A:** PO, rapidly absorbed from GI tract • **M:** Extensively metabolized • **E:** Renal excretion	**MOA:** • Blocks viral uncoating • Longer half-life than amantadine	• Influenza treatment	• Lower risk of CNS adverse effects than amantadine
Guanosine Analogs				
Ribavirin (Virazole)	• **A:** PO, inhaled, and IV; PO absorption increased with high fat meals and decreased with coingestion of antacids • **E:** Parent drug and metabolites excreted in urine	**MOA:** • Inhibits synthesis of GTP • Inhibits viral RNA-dependent RNA polymerase • Inhibits capping of viral mRNA	• Aerosolized form for influenza treatment • Aerosolized treatment of bronchiolitis caused by respiratory syncytial virus • Keratitis due to herpes • IV treatment decreases mortality if used early in Lassa fever • Treatment of hepatitis C (with interferon)	• Contraindicated in pregnancy: known teratogen • Systemic use results in dose-dependent myelosuppression • Aerosol may cause conjunctival or bronchial irritation • Psychiatric side effects (depression and suicidal behavior)

Glycoproteins

Interferon-alfa (Alferon N, Roferon, and Intron) Interferon-beta (Avonex, Betaseron)	• **A:** IV, SC, or IM	**MOA:** • Endogenous proteins with multiple mechanisms of action that exert antiviral, immunoregulatory, and antiproliferative activities	• Chronic hepatitis C • Chronic myelogenous leukemia • Malignant myeloma • Hairy cell leukemia, • AIDS-related Kaposi's sarcoma • Genital warts • Relapsing multiple sclerosis	• Neutropenia • Anemia • Thrombocytopenia • Elevated aminotransferase levels • Flu-like symptoms • Nausea • Diarrhea

Pyrophosphanate Derivative

Foscarnet (Foscavir)	• **A:** IV • **D:** Good penetration into tissues; crosses BBB; CNS concentration is ~50% of serum concentration • **E:** Majority excreted unchanged in urine	**MOA:** • Directly inhibits viral RNA and DNA polymerases and HIV reverse transcriptase by interacting with the pyrophosphate binding site **Resistance:** • Via point mutations in the DNA polymerase gene	• CMV retinitis, colitis, and esophagitis • Acyclovir-resistant HSV infection • Acyclovir-resistant VZV infection	• More expensive and less well tolerated than ganciclovir • Renal insufficiency • Hypocalcemia or hypercalcemia • Hypophosphatemia or hyperphosphatemia • Penile ulcerations due to high drug concentrations in urine • CNS (eg, headache, hallucinations, seizures)

MAJOR SITES OF DRUG ACTION ON VIRAL REPLICATION

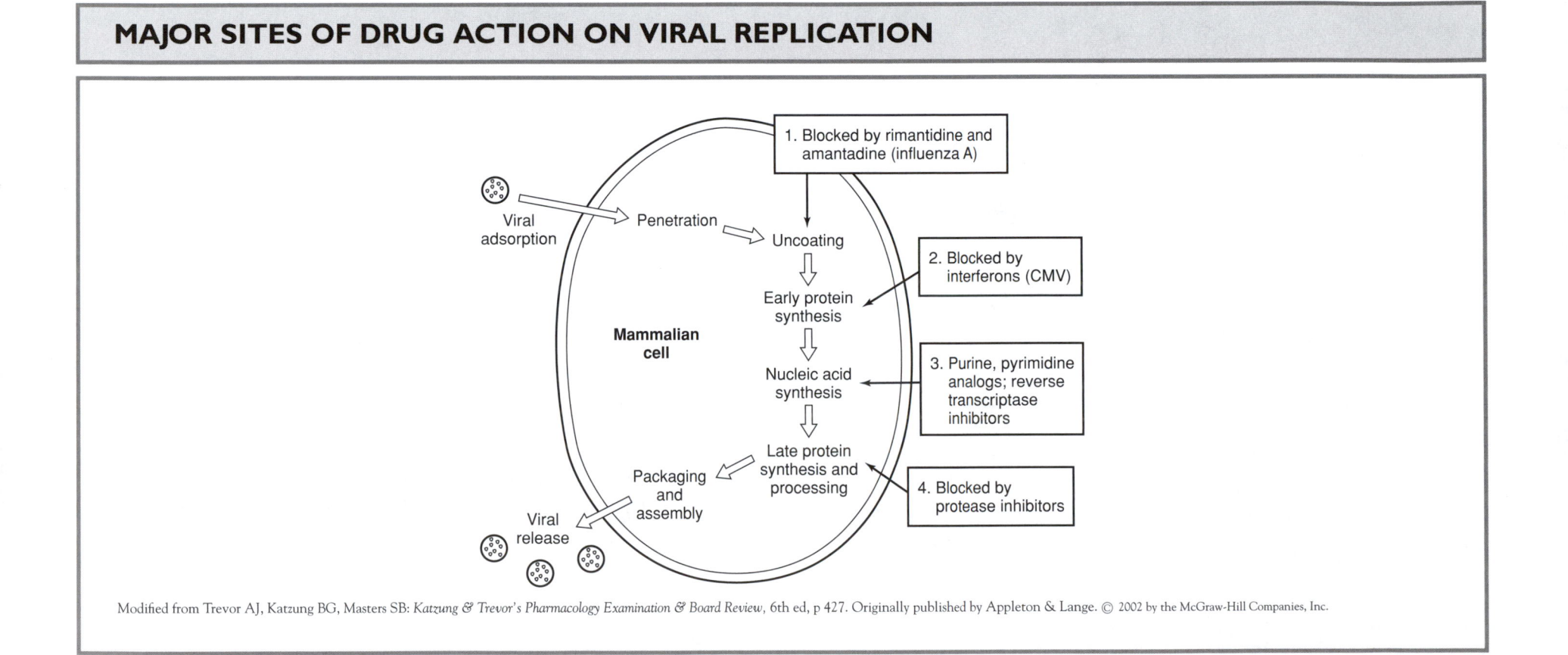

Modified from Trevor AJ, Katzung BG, Masters SB: *Katzung & Trevor's Pharmacology Examination & Board Review*, 6th ed, p 427. Originally published by Appleton & Lange. © 2002 by the McGraw-Hill Companies, Inc.

NUCLEOSIDE ANALOGUES

Drug	Pharmacokinetics	Mechanisms of Action and of Resistance	Clinical Uses	Drawbacks and Side Effects
Acyclovir (Zovirax)	• **A:** PO, IV, and topical • **D:** Well distributed; crosses BBB; CSF concentration 50% of serum concentration • **E:** Majority excreted unchanged in urine	**MOA:** • First phosphorylation by viral thymidine kinase • Second and third phosphorylations by host cell kinases • Acyclovir-triphosphate is then incorporated into viral DNA causing premature termination **Resistance:** • Via alteration in viral thymidine kinase • Via alteration in DNA polymerase • Confers cross resistance to valacyclovir, famciclovir, and ganciclovir	• Primary or recurrent genital herpes • HSV encephalitis or neonatal HSV infection • HSV lesions	• Nausea • Diarrhea • Headache • IV infusion associated with renal insufficiency or CNS toxicity (tremors or delirium)
Valacyclovir (Valtrex)	• **A:** PO • **M:** Rapidly converted to acyclovir following hepatic metabolism; produces serum levels 3–5 times those achieved with PO acyclovir • **E:** Metabolite excreted in urine	**MOA:** • First phosphorylation by viral thymidine kinase • Second and third phosphorylations by host cell kinases • Acyclovir-triphosphate is then incorporated into viral DNA causing premature termination	• Primary or recurrent genital herpes as well as prophylaxis • Herpes zoster infection • Prevention of CMV following organ transplantation	• Nausea • Diarrhea • Headache

Continued

NUCLEOSIDE ANALOGUES (Continued)

Drug	Pharmacokinetics	Mechanisms of Action and of Resistance	Clinical Uses	Drawbacks and Side Effects
Ganciclovir (Cytovene)	• **A:** IV for acute treatment; PO for maintenance therapy (bioavailability <10%); ophthalmic • **D:** Well distributed; crosses BBB; CSF concentration 50% of serum concentration • **E:** Unchanged in urine	**MOA:** • First phosphorylation by viral thymidine kinase • Triphosphorylated form inhibits DNA polymerases of CMV and HSV **Resistance:** • Via alteration in viral kinase	• CMV retinitis, colitis, or esophagitis in HIV patients • CMV prophylaxis in HIV patients	• Systemic treatment can lead to myelosuppression • Rare CNS toxicity (seizures)
Trifluridine (Viroptic)	• **A:** Topical	**MOA:** • Phosphorylated by cellular enzymes • Active form inhibits viral DNA synthesis	• Drug of choice for keratoconjunctivitis due to HSV-1 or HSV-2 • Acyclovir-resistant HSV infections	• Limited because of topical administration • Too toxic for systemic use
Vidarabine (Vira-A)	• **A:** Topical	**MOA:** • Phosphorylated by intracellular enzymes • Activated form inhibits viral DNA polymerase	• Keratitis due to herpes	• Limited because of topical administration • Systemic treatment associated with GI irritation, paresthesias, tremor, convulsions, hepatic dysfunction

NUCLEOSIDE REVERSE TRANSCRIPTASE INHIBITORS

Drug	Pharmacokinetics	Mechanisms of Action and of Resistance	Clinical Uses	Drawbacks and Side Effects
Zidovudine/ AZT/ZDV (Retrovir)	• **A:** PO and IV • **D:** Widely distributed; CNS concentration is 60% of plasma concentration • **M:** Rapidly undergoes hepatic glucuronidation • **E:** Parent drug and metabolites excreted in urine	**MOA:** • Phosphorylated to form a nucleotide analog by cellular kinases • Inhibits reverse transcriptase of HIV-1 and HIV-2 • Causes chain termination • Reverse transcriptase is more susceptible to inhibitory effect of these than mammalian DNA polymerase **Resistance:** • Develops rapidly with monotherapy	• HIV treatment • Often used with lamivudine (3TC) • Reduces vertical transmission to fetus • Palliative treatment (only can eliminate active virus)	• Bone marrow suppression • Headache • Nausea • Insomnia • Myalgias • Severe neurotoxicity • Rare occurrences of fatal lactic acidosis and severe hepatomegaly with steatosis **Drug interactions:** • Drugs that inhibit glucuronidation • Drugs metabolized by liver • Antineoplastics and nephrotoxic drugs
Didanosine/ ddI (Videx)	• **A:** PO; must be taken on an empty stomach (acid inhibits absorption) • **D:** CSF concentrations are ~20% of serum concentrations • **E:** In urine via glomerular filtration and tubular secretion	**MOA:** • Activated by cellular kinases • Phosphorylated for inhibits reverse transcriptase and causes chain termination **Resistance:** • Confers cross resistance to abacavir, ddC, and 3TC	• HIV treatment • Often used with d4T	• Peripheral neuropathy • Pancreatitis • Diarrhea • Hyperuricemia • Cardiomyopathy • CNS toxicity • Rare occurrences of fatal lactic acidosis and severe hepatomegaly with steatosis

Continued

NUCLEOSIDE REVERSE TRANSCRIPTASE INHIBITORS (Continued)

Drug	Pharmacokinetics	Mechanisms of Action and of Resistance	Clinical Uses	Drawbacks and Side Effects
Zalcitabine/ ddC (HIVID)	• **A:** PO; high bioavailability, antacids and food decrease absorption • **D:** CNS concentration only 20% of serum concentration • **E:** Majority excreted unchanged in urine	**MOA:** • Inhibits reverse transcriptase	• HIV treatment • Used in combination therapy to avoid drug resistance	• Headache • Fever • Peripheral neuropathy • Pancreatitis • Rare occurrences of fatal lactic acidosis and severe hepatomegaly with steatosis **Drug interactions:** • Not good with ddI, d4T, and INH (similar side effects); amphotericin B, foscarnet, and aminoglycosides • Increase risk of peripheral neuropathy
Lamivudine/ 3TC (Epivir)	• **A:** PO; high bioavailability • **E:** Unchanged in urine	**MOA:** • Phosphorylated by host cell kinases • Inhibits reverse transcriptase **Resistance:** • Confers cross resistance to abacavir, ddI, and ddC	• HIV treatment • Chronic hepatitis B treatment	• Headache • Insomnia • Fatigue • GI distress

Stavudine/d4T (Zerit)	• **A:** PO; high bioavailability • **D:** CSF concentration is 55% of serum concentration • **E:** In urine via active tubular secretion and glomerular filtration	**MOA:** • Inhibits reverse transcriptase **Resistance:** • Confers cross resistance to ddI and ddC	• HIV treatment • Convenient for use in HIV patients because it can be taken without regard to meals only twice daily • Used with ddI or 3TC	• Sensory neuropathy • Pancreatitis • Headache • Nausea • Rare occurrences of fatal lactic acidosis when used with other antiretroviral agents in pregnant women **Drug interactions:** • Amphotericin, foscarnet, dapsone, and other drugs increase risk of peripheral neuropathy • Reduces phosphorylation of ZDV therefore they are not used together
Abacavir (Ziagen)	• **A:** PO • **M:** Hepatic metabolism • **E:** Metabolites excreted in urine and feces	**MOA:** • Active metabolite is incorporated into viral DNA where it prevents viral DNA elongation and inhibits the activity of HIV reverse transcriptase **Resistance:** • Confers resistance to 3TC, ddI, and ddC	• HIV treatment	• Hypersensitivity • Hepatotoxicity • Lactic acidosis • Pancreatitis

NON–NUCLEOSIDE REVERSE TRANSCRIPTASE INHIBITORS

Drug	Pharmacokinetics	Mechanisms of Action and of Resistance	Clinical Uses and General Information	Drawbacks and Side Effects
Nevirapine (Viramune)	• **A:** PO, high bioavailability • **B:** 60% protein bound • **D:** CSF concentration 45% of serum concentration • **M:** Extensive hepatic metabolism by P450 enzymes • **E:** Metabolites excreted in urine	**MOA:** • Inhibit reverse transcriptase **Resistance:** • Via mutations in the *pol* gene, which encodes for reverse transcriptase	• HIV treatment • Can be combined with NRTIs for HIV treatment • Allows protease inhibitors to be saved for later treatment	• Resistance develops rapidly with monotherapy • Hypersensitivity reactions include Stevens-Johnson syndrome and life-threatening toxic epidermal necrolysis **Drug interactions:** • With drugs that act on the P450 enzymes
Delavirdine (Rescriptor)	• **A:** PO, high bioavailability • **B:** 98% protein bound • **D:** Low CSF levels • **M:** Hepatic metabolism by P450 enzymes to inactive metabolites • **E:** Metabolites excreted in feces and urine			• Resistance develops rapidly with monotherapy • Skin rash • Headache • Fatigue • Nausea • Diarrhea • A known teratogen in animals, so avoid in pregnant women **Drug interactions:** • With drugs that act on the P450 enzymes
Efavirenz (Sustiva)	• **A:** PO • **M:** Hepatic metabolism by P450 enzymes • **E:** Unchanged drug excreted in feces, metabolites excreted in urine			• Resistance develops rapidly with monotherapy • Depression • Skin rash • Hematuria • Renal calculi

PROTEASE INHIBITORS

Drug	Pharmacokinetics	Mechanisms of Action and of Resistance	Clinical Uses	Drawbacks and Side Effects
Indinavir (Crixivan)	• **A:** PO; should be taken on empty stomach due to improved absorption under acidic conditions; good bioavailability • **M:** Hepatic metabolized by P450 system • **E:** Metabolites excreted in feces	**MOA:** • Inhibit viral protease that cleaves precursor proteins **Resistance:** • Via mutations in the *pol* gene, which encodes for reverse transcriptase • Confers cross resistance to class members	• HIV treatment • Can be used alone (resistance will develop) • Usually used in combination with nucleoside analogue	• Nausea • Diarrhea • Hyperbilirubinemia • Nephrolithiasis **Drug interactions:** • With drugs that act on the P450 enzymes
Saquinavir (Invirase, Fortovase)	• **A:** PO; low bioavailability, improved when taken with food • **B:** 98% protein bound • **M:** Hepatic metabolism by P450 enzymes • **E:** Metabolites excreted in feces			• GI distress • Rhinitis • Headache • Neutropenia **Drug interactions:** • With drugs that act on the P450 enzymes
Ritonavir (Norvir)	• **A:** PO; good bioavailability, improved when taken with meals • **M:** Hepatic metabolism • **E:** Metabolites excreted in feces			• GI distress • Paresthesias • Hypertriglyceridemia **Drug interactions:** • With drugs that act on the P450 enzymes
Amprenavir (Agenerase)	• **A:** PO • **M:** Hepatic metabolism by P450 enzymes • **E:** Majority of metabolites excreted in feces; remainder in urine			• Hyperglycemia • Skin rash (including Stevens-Johnson syndrome) • Mood disorders **Drug interactions:** • With drugs that act on the P450 enzymes

VI. Antifungal Agents

MECHANISMS OF ACTION AND CLASSIFICATION OF ANTIFUNGAL AGENTS

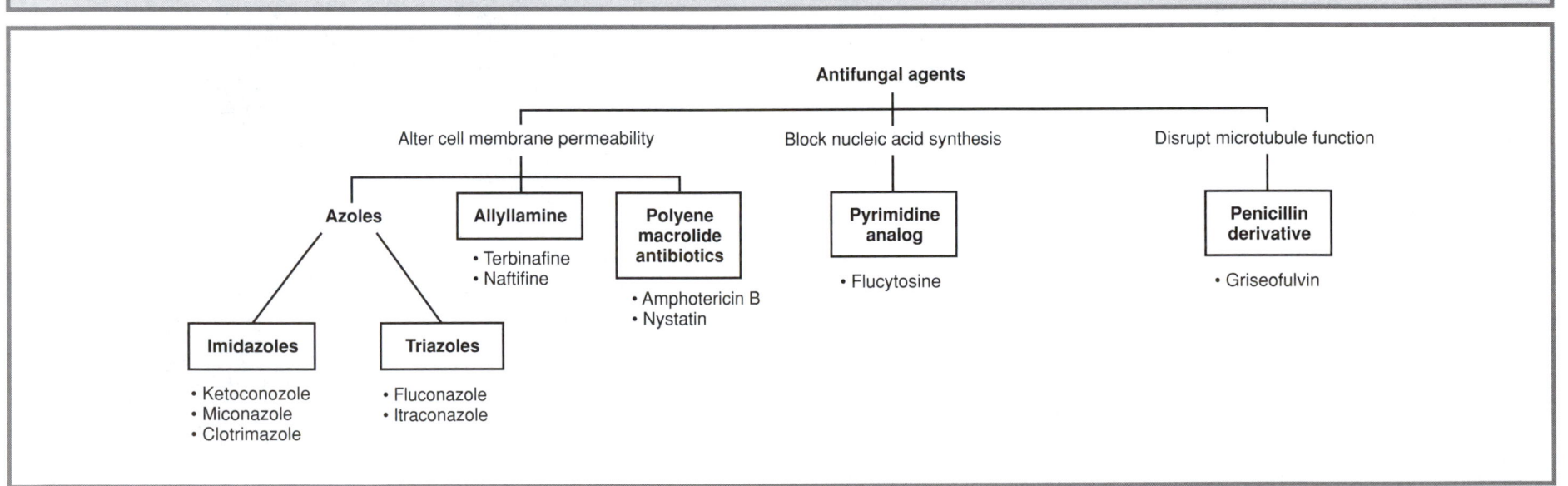

FUNGAL INFECTIONS ACCORDING TO COMMONESS

Most common	Cutaneous (skin, hair, nails, tinea cruris)
Common	Mucocutaneous (GI, perianal, oral)
Least common	Systemic (invasive aspergillosis, cryptococcal meningitis, pulmonary histoplasmosis) • Potentially life-threatening infections in immunocompromised patients

ANTIFUNGALS: DRUG FACTS

Drug	Pharmacokinetics	Mechanisms of Action and of Resistance	Spectrum of Activity	Clinical Uses and General Information	Drawbacks and Side Effects
Polyene Macrolide Antibiotics					
Amphotericin B (Amphotec, Fungizone)	• **A:** IV (major use); PO, good for luminal gut infections due to poor absorption; topical • **B:** 90% protein binding • **D:** Does not penetrate BBB • **E:** Via hepatic metabolism	**MOA:** • Bind to sterols (especially ergosterol) in cell membrane forming cytotoxic pores **Resistance:** • Via decreased membrane concentration of egosterol • Via modification of sterol binding site	• Broadest spectrum of all antifungals • *Candida albicans* • *Cryptococcus neoformans* • *Aspergillus* • *Histoplasma capsulatum* • *Blastomyces dermatitidis*	• Systemic infections • Fungal meningitis • Dermatophytic infections • Mucocutaneous infections	• Infusion hypersensitivity reactions (nausea, vomiting, chills, hypotension) • Nephrotoxicity • Hypokalemia • Hypomagnesemia • Arrhythmias
Nystatin (Mycostatin)	• **A:** Topical and PO; poorly absorbed		• *C albicans*	• Mucocutaneous candidal infections	• Local topical reactions • Too dangerous for systemic administration
Pyrimidine Analog					
Flucytosine (Ancobon)	• **A:** PO • **D:** Widely distributed; crosses BBB • **E:** 80% is excreted unchanged in urine via glomerular filtration	**MOA:** • Incorporated into nucleic acids and inhibits fungal DNA and RNA synthesis **Resistance:** • Via altered metabolism of flucytosine • Develops rapidly with monotherapy	• *C neoformans* • Some candidal species • Dermatiaceous molds	• Always in combination therapy with another drug • With amphotericin B for cryptococcal meningitis • With itraconazole for chromoblastomycosis	• Narrow therapeutic window • Alopecia • Enterocolitis • Bone marrow toxicity (anemia, thrombocytopenia, and leukopenia) • Hepatotoxic

Continued

ANTIFUNGALS: DRUG FACTS (Continued)

Drug	Pharmacokinetics	Mechanisms of Action and of Resistance	Spectrum of Activity	Clinical Uses and General Information	Drawbacks and Side Effects
Penicillin Derivative					
Griseofulvin (Grifulvin, Grisactin)	• **A:** PO; fatty meals enhance absorption • **M:** Hepatic metabolism • **E:** Metabolites excreted in urine and feces	**MOA:** • Inhibits fungal cell mitosis by disrupting microtubules in mitotic spindle • May also inhibit synthesis of nucleic acids • Binds to keratin in newly forming skin, hair, and nails **Resistance:** • Via decrease in energy dependent transport of the drug into the dermatophyte	• Dermatophytes	• Systemic treatment of dermatophytic infections	• Lethargy, insomnia, fatigue • Hepatitis **Drug Interactions:** • Warfarin • Phenobarbital
Imidazoles					
Ketoconazole (Nizoral)	• **A:** Topical and PO; absorption is low but improves with food due to low gastric pH • **D:** Does not cross BBB • **M:** Hepatic metabolism • **E:** Parent drug and metabolites excreted in feces and urine	**MOA:** • Inhibit synthesis of ergosterol	• *C neoformans* • Numerous candidal species • Endemic mycoses (*Blastomyces*, *Coccidioides*, and *Histoplasma*) • Dermatophytes	• Back-up drug for systemic infections caused by *Blastomyces*, *Coccidioides*, and *Histoplasma* • Mucocutaneous candidiasis • Non-meningeal coccidioidomycosis • Seborrheic dermatitis (shampoo preparation) • Pityriasis versicolor	• Narrow therapeutic window • Inhibition of mammalian P450 microsomal enzymes (numerous drug interactions) • Nausea and vomiting • Adrenal and gonadal steroid synthesis inhibition • Resistance increasing in incidence especially with prophylactic use

Miconazole (Monistat)	• **A:** Topical and IV	• Numerous candidal species • Dermatophytes	• Available over the counter • Vulvovaginal candidiasis • Dermatophytic infections (tinea cruris, tinea corporis, and tinea pedis)	• Rare • Resistance increasing in incidence especially with prophylactic use
Clotrimazole (Mycelex, Gyne-Lotrimin)	• **A:** Topical		• Available over the counter • Vulvovaginal candidiasis • Dermatophytic infections (tinea cruris, tinea corporis, and tinea pedis) • Oropharyngeal thrush (better tasting than nystatin)	

Continued

ANTIFUNGALS: DRUG FACTS (Continued)

Drug	Pharmacokinetics	Mechanisms of Action and of Resistance	Spectrum of Activity	Clinical Uses and General Information	Drawbacks and Side Effects
Triazoles					
Fluconazole (Diflucan)	• **A:** PO and IV; good absorption • **D:** Crosses BBB • **E:** Unchanged in urine	See page 58.	• Numerous candidal species • *C neoformans*	• Drug of choice for mucocutaneous candidiasis • Prophylaxis and treatment of cryptococcal meningitis • Single dose for vaginal candidiasis • Prophylactically for bone marrow transplant patients and AIDS patients • Least risk of this family for drug interactions due to low effect on hepatic microsomal enzymes	• Resistance increasing in incidence especially with prophylactic use

Itraconazole (Sporanox)	• **A:** PO and IV; low bioavailability is improved with food due to decreased gastric pH • **D:** Does not cross BBB • **M:** Metabolized by hepatic P450 enzymes • **E:** Majority of metabolites excreted in urine		• *Aspergillus* • Dermatophytes • Endemic mycoses (*Histoplasma, Blastomyces,* and *Sporothrix*)	• Most potent of azole antifungals for systemic infection • Drug of choice for dermatophytoses and onychomycosis • Only drug effective against *Aspergillus* infections • Preferred agent for endemic mycosis (*Histoplasma, Blastomyces,* and *Sporothrix*)	• Less affect on hepatic microsomal enzymes than ketoconazole; therefore, less risk of drug interactions than ketoconazole • Resistance increasing in incidence especially with prophylactic use

Allyllamine

Terbinafine (Lamisil)	• **A:** Topical and PO	• Inhibits fungal metabolism of squalene leading to accumulation of toxic levels of squalene	• Dermatophytes	• Treatment of dermatophytoses especially onychomycosis	• Rare • GI upset • Headache
Naftifine (Naftin)	• **A:** Topical				• Rare

VII. Antiprotozoal Agents

THERAPEUTIC CLASSIFICATION OF ANTIPROTOZOAL AGENTS

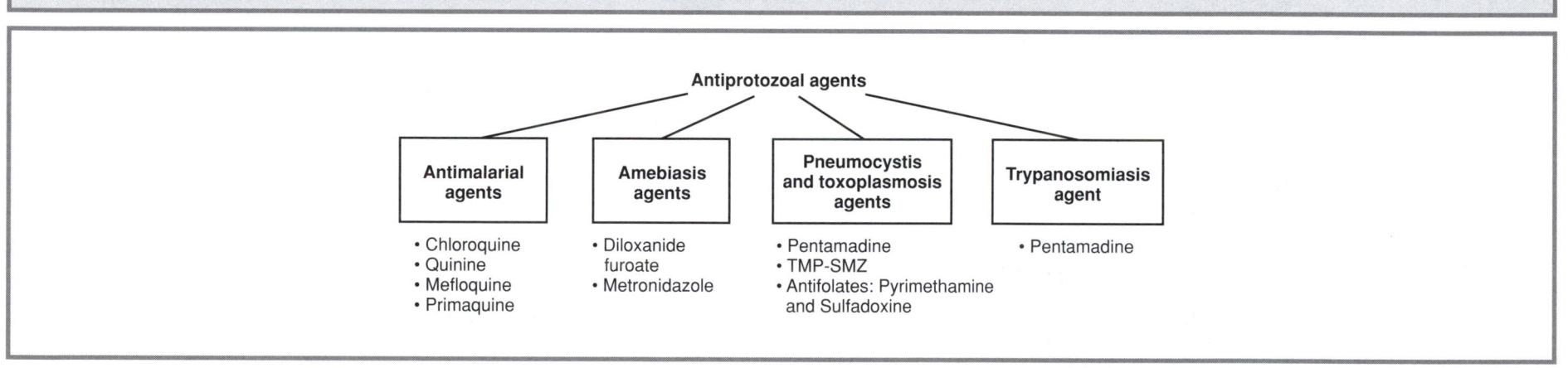

THERAPEUTIC APPLICATIONS OF ANTIPROTOZOAL DRUGS

Disease	Drugs	Clinical Uses	Memory Tools ☞
Malaria	Chloroquine	Drug of choice in acute attacks	Spread by female mosquito, so think—**make the queen fall 4 times** or **quin fol**
	Quinine	Used for strains resistant to chloroquine	
	Mefloquine	For prophylaxis	
	Primaquine	Not for acute attacks but is used for liver stages of malarial life cycle	
	Antifols	Not used for prophylaxis	
Amebiasis	Diloxanide furoate	Asymptomatic intestinal infection	**AID: A**symptomatic **I**ntestinal **D**iloxanide
	Metronidazole plus iodoquinol or diloxanide	Mild to severe intestinal infection	**MILD**
	Metronidazole plus Diloxanide, followed by Chloroquine	Hepatic Abscess	**HAM, Dill Pickle & Chips**
Toxoplasmosis	Pyrimethamine plus sulfadiazine	Combination of choice	Often transmitted to humans via cat feces. Visualize a cat who purrs: **Pyr + s**
Pneumocystis carinii pneumonia	Trimethoprim-sulfamethoxazole (TMP-SMZ)	Drug combination of choice	*P carinii* pneumonia is abbreviated PCP, so TMP-SMZ rhymes with PCP
	Pentamadine	Alternative therapy	
	Atovaquone	Less effective, but better tolerated; used for mild to moderate PCP	

ANTIPROTOZOALS: DRUG FACTS

Drug	Pharmacokinetics	Mechanisms of Action and of Resistance	Clinical Uses and General Information	Drawbacks and Side Effects
Chloroquine (Aralen)	• **A:** IM, IV, SC, PO (best); absorption is rapid and complete from GI tract • **D:** Widely distributed • **E:** Parent drug and metabolites excreted in urine	**MOA:** • Prevents polymerization of hemoglobin breakdown product, heme, into hemozoin • Intracellular accumulation of heme is toxic to parasite **Resistance:** • Via expulsion of the drug by a bacterial pump	• Drug of choice for treatment and prophylaxis of malaria • Used to treat erythrocytic stage of *Plasmodium infections* • Combined with metronidazole to treat amebic liver disease • Also used to treat autoimmune disorders • Resistance common with *Plasmodium falciparum* infection • Some resistance in *Plasmodium vivax*	**Associated with low dose:** • Nausea and vomiting • Dizziness • Blurring of vision • Headache • Skin rash **Associated with high dose:** • Retinopathies • Psychosis • Myocardial depression
Quinine	• **A:** IV; PO, rapidly absorbed • **M:** Hepatic metabolism • **E:** Parent drug and metabolites excreted in urine	**MOA:** • Complexes with double-stranded DNA to prevent strand separation • Blocks DNA replication and transcription to RNA	• Treatment of chloroquine-resistant *P falciparum* • Effective against all erythrocytic forms of malaria • Gametocidal for *P vivax* and *Plasmodium ovale*	• Cinchonism • Hemolysis in patients with G6PD deficiency • Blackwater fever • Should be avoided in patients with underlying auditory or visual problems

Mefloquine (Lariam)	**A:** PO **M:** Hepatic metabolism **E:** Drug and metabolites excreted in feces	**MOA:** • Unknown	• Malaria prophylaxis • Active against erythrocytic stage of *P vivax* and *P falciparum*	• GI distress • Skin rash • Headache • Dizziness • Can precipitate seizures or neurologic symptoms • Can precipitate cardiac conduction abnormalities, especially when combined with drugs such as quinidine or β-blockers • Contraindicated in patients with history of epilepsy or psychiatric disorders
Primaquine	**A:** PO; daily doses required **M:** Hepatic metabolism **E:** Parent drug and metabolites excreted in urine	**MOA:** • Forms quinoline-quinone metabolites, electron-transferring redox compounds that act as cellular oxidants • Acts as a tissue schizonticide	• Treatment of liver stages of *P vivax* and *P ovale* • Prophylaxis for exposed individuals • Used with clindamycin to treat pneumocystosis	• GI distress • Pruritus • Headaches • Methemoglobinemia • Hemolysis in patients with G6PD deficiency

Continued

ANTIPROTOZOALS: DRUG FACTS (Continued)

Drug	Pharmacokinetics	Mechanisms of Action and of Resistance	Clinical Uses and General Information	Drawbacks and Side Effects
Pyrimethamine and sulfadoxine (Fansidar)	• **A:** PO • **D:** Penetrate CNS well • **E:** Partly unchanged in urine	**MOA:** • Both drugs act synergistically to inhibit folate synthesis, which is required for DNA synthesis • Pyrimethamine inhibits dihydrofolate reductase • Sulfadoxine inhibits dihydropteroate synthase	• Primarily active against erythrocytic forms of malaria • Some activity against primary *Plasmodium* infection in the liver • Pyrimethamine is used with sulfadiazine for treatment of toxoplasmosis	**Pyrimethamine:** • Skin rashes • Pruritus • GI upset **Sulfadoxine:** • Fever • Skin rash (Stevens-Johnson syndrome ≈1%) • GI upset • Hemolysis • Nephrotoxicity
Metronidazole (Flagyl)	• **A:** PO • **M:** Hepatic • **E:** Parent drug and metabolites excreted in urine	**MOA:** • Forms cytotoxic products via reductive bioactivation of its nitro group • Causes oxidative damage to DNA of trophozoite	• Most effective drug against invasive form of *Entamoeba histolytica* • Drug of choice for giardiasis, trichomoniasis, *Gardnerella vaginalis* infections, and infections caused by anaerobic bacteria	• GI distress • Headache • Dry mouth • Metallic taste • Disulfiram reaction (nausea and vomiting with coingestion of alcohol)
Diloxanide furoate (Furamide, Entamide)	• **A:** PO; 90% unabsorbed, which makes it an effective luminal amebicide	**MOA:** • Unknown	• Asymptomatic amebiasis • Luminal amebicide • Severe cases of amebiasis require both types of amebicides (intestinal and extraintestinal acting agents)	• GI distress (nausea and abdominal cramps)

Iodoquinol (Diquinol, Yodoxin)	• **A:** PO • **E:** Majority excreted unchanged in feces	**MOA:** • Unknown	• Luminal amebicide	• Peripheral neuropathy • Visual dysfunction
Trimethoprim-Sulfamethoxazole (TMP-SMZ) (Bactrim, Septra)	• **A:** PO; rapidly absorbed • **M:** Hepatic • **E:** Parent drug and metabolites excreted in urine	**MOA:** • Both drugs act synergistically to inhibit folate synthesis, which is required for DNA synthesis	• Prophylaxis and treatment of PCP in AIDS patients • Prophylaxis of toxoplasmosis in AIDS patients	• GI distress • Rash • Photosensitivity • Renal failure • Hepatitis • Neutropenia • Thrombocytopenia • Stevens-Johnson syndrome
Pentamidine (Pentam 300, Pentacarinat)	• **A:** IM, IV, and aerosol • **E:** Majority of drug eliminated slowly in urine	**MOA:** • Unknown • May inhibit glycolysis or may interfere with nucleic acid metabolism in fungi	• Trypanosomiasis • Aerosolized form for pneumocystosis or toxoplasmosis prophylaxis	• Respiratory stimulation then depression • Hypotension • Hypoglycemia • Anemia and neutropenia • Hepatitis • Pancreatitis
Atovaquone (Mepron)	• **A:** PO • **E:** In feces	**MOA:** • Inhibits mitochondrial electron transport	• Treatment and prophylaxis of PCP • Treatment and prophylaxis of toxoplasmosis	• Rash • Cough • Nausea, vomiting, diarrhea • Fever • Abnormal LFTs

VIII. Antihelminthic Agents

ANTIHELMINTHICS: DRUG FACTS

Drug	Pharmacokinetics	Mechanisms of Action	Clinical Use	Drawbacks and Side Effects
Mebendozole (Vermox)	• **A:** PO; poorly absorbed • **B:** >90% protein bound • **M:** Rapidly metabolized • **E:** Most in urine (small amount in bile)	• Inhibits microtubule synthesis and glucose uptake in nematodes	• Pinworm infections • Whipworm infections	• GI distress • Contraindicated during pregnancy
Pyrantel pamoate (Antiminth, Combantrin)	• **A:** PO; poorly absorbed • **E:** Parent drug and metabolites excreted in urine; unabsorbed drug excreted in feces	• Depolarizing neuromuscular blocker, which causes paralysis of nematodes	• Hookworm infections • Pinworm infections • Roundworm infections	• GI distress • Headache • Weakness
Praziquantel (Biltricide)	• **A:** PO; rapidly absorbed • **M:** Extensive first pass hepatic metabolism • **E:** Mainly in urine (small amount in feces)	• Increases membrane permeability to Ca^+ causing muscular contraction and paralysis of the trematode muscles • Eventually causes vacuolization and death	• Drug of choice for schistosomiasis, clonorchiasis, and paragonimiasis • Treatment of infections caused by small and large intestinal flukes • Tapeworm infections • Cysticercosis	• GI distress • Headache • Malaise • Rash • Fever
Niclosamide (Niclocide)	• **A:** PO; poorly absorbed • **E:** In feces	• Unknown • May act by uncoupling oxidative phosphorylation or by activating ATPases • Acts against cestodes	• Infections from ingestion of beef, pork, and fish • Infections caused by small and large intestinal flukes	• GI distress • Headache • Rash • Fever

IX. Antimycobacterial Agents

AVAILABLE AGENTS FOR TUBERCULOSIS AND LEPROSY PLUS ATYPICAL MYCOBACTERIAL AGENTS

First-line agents for treating tuberculosis include the following:
Rifampin
Ethambutol
Streptomycin
Pyrazinamide
Isoniazid
☞ **RESPI**ration

Second-line agents for tuberculosis include the following:
Amikacin
Capreomycin
Ciprofloxacin/**L**evofloxacin
p-**A**minosalicylic acid
Cycloserine
Ethionamide
Rifabutin
☞ **A**ll these **C**an **C**lear **L**ungs **A**nd **C**an **E**ase **R**espiration

Agents for treating leprosy include the following:
Dapsone
Clofazamine
Rifampin
   for
Leprosy
☞ **D**rugs **C**an **R**emove **L**esions

Agents that are classified as atypical mycobacterial drugs include the following:
Macrolide **A**ntibiotics
Rifabutin
Tetracyclines
☞ **MART**

ANTIMYCOBACTERIALS: DRUG FACTS

Drug	Pharmacokinetics	Mechanisms of Action and of Resistance	Clinical Uses and General Information	Drawbacks and Side Effects
Isoniazid (INH) ☞ **INH** **I**nhibits mycolic acid synthesis **N**europathy **H**epatotoxicity	• **A:** IM and PO; well absorbed • **D:** Well distributed; crosses BBB • **M:** Hepatic acetylation (note that rate of acetylation is genetically determined) • **E:** In urine	**MOA:** • Inhibits the synthesis of mycolic acids • Mycolic acids are essential components of the mycobacterial cell wall • Tuburculocidal to intracellular and extracelluar organisms **Resistance:** • Via mutation in the gene coding for the enzyme required for drug activation	• Most active of all anti-TB drugs • First-line of treatment in multidrug combination for TB • Single agent prophylaxis for skin test converters and high risk populations • Not effective against *Mycobacterium kansasii* and *Mycobacterium avium-intracellulare* complex	• Allergic reactions • Hepatitis • Peripheral neuropathy (increased risk in slow acetylator populations) • Lupus-like syndrome • CNS toxicity (memory loss, insomnia, and seizures) • Hemolysis in patients with G6PD deficiency • Drug resistance emerges rapidly with monotherapy
Rifampin (Rifadin) ☞ 4 R's for Rifampin: **R**evs up P450 **R**NA polymerase inhibitor **R**ed/orange bodily fluids **R**apid resistance if used alone	• **A:** IV and PO; well absorbed • **B:** Highly protein bound • **D:** Only crosses inflamed meninges • **M:** Rapid hepatic metabolism • **E:** Metabolites excreted in feces; parent drug and metabolites excreted in urine	**MOA:** • Inhibits RNA synthesis by binding to the β subunit of DNA-dependent RNA polymerase in susceptible microorganisms • Inhibits protein synthesis by preventing chain initiation • Virtually no effect on mammalian RNA polymerase • Tuberculocidal to intracellular and extracellular organisms **Resistance:** • Via mutation in gene coding for β subunit of DNA-dependent RNA polymerase	• First-line of treatment in multidrug combination for TB • First-line of treatment in multidrug combination for leprosy • Also used for a variety of other diseases including prophylaxis for meningococcal meningitis	• Causes orange-colored urine, tears, sweat, and contact lenses • Induces microsomal enzymes (drug interactions) • Rashes • Fever • Thrombocytopenia • Nausea and vomiting • Hepatotoxicity • Drug resistance develops rapidly with monotherapy

Ethambutol (Myambutol)	• **A:** PO; well absorbed • **D:** Widely distributed; only crosses inflamed meninges • **E:** Unchanged in urine and feces	**MOA:** • Inhibits arabinosyl transferase, an enzyme in the synthesis of arabinogalactan (a component of mycobacterium cell wall) • Tuberculostatic to intracellular and extracellular organisms **Resistance:** • Via mutation in the gene coding for the arabinosyl transferase	• First-line treatment of TB in combination with INH or rifampin	• Hypersensitivity (rare) • Optic neuritis (precludes use in children too young for visual examinations) • Drug resistance develops rapidly with monotherapy
Pyrazinamide (PZA, Tebrazid)	• **A:** PO; well absorbed • **D:** Widely distributed; only crosses inflamed meninges • **M:** Hepatic metabolism • **E:** Majority of metabolites excreted in urine	**MOA:** • Precise MOA unknown • Requires enzymatic activation • Acts in macrophages • Tuberculocidal only to intracellular organisms **Resistance:** • Via lack of activating enzymes • Via decreased drug uptake	• First-line, short-term treatment in multidrug combination for TB • With ofloxacin or ciprofloxacin to prevent active disease in high risk populations exposed to multidrug-resistant TB	• Hepatotoxicity • Nongouty polyarthralgia • Hyperuricemia (may precipitate gout) • Myalgia • GI irritation • Porphyria • Drug resistance develops rapidly with monotherapy
Streptomycin	• **A:** IM; good • **D:** Widely distributed; enters CNS only with inflamed meninges • **E:** In urine	**MOA:** • Irreversibly blocks bacterial protein synthesis by binding to the 30S ribosomal subunit • Tuberculocidal only to extracellular organisms (poor for intracellular organisms)	• Second- and third-line in multidrug combination to treat TB resistant to first-line drugs • Indicated for severe TB: disseminating disease and meningitis	• Ototoxicity • Nephrotoxicity • Drug resistance precludes monotherapy

Continued

ANTIMYCOBACTERIALS: DRUG FACTS (Continued)

Drug	Pharmacokinetics	Mechanisms of Action and of Resistance	Clinical Uses and General Information	Drawbacks and Side Effects
Amikacin (Amikin)	• **A:** IM or IV • **E:** In urine unchanged	**MOA:** • Blocks bacterial protein synthesis by binding to the 30S ribosomal subunit	• Second-line drug for TB treatment • Indicated for use with streptomycin-resistant or multidrug-resistant TB (most remain susceptible) • Active against atypical mycobacterium as well • Used in combination drug regimens to avoid emergence of resistance	• Ototoxic • Nephrotoxic
Capreomycin (Capastat)	• **A:** IM and IV • **E:** Majority excreted unchanged in urine	**MOA:** • Peptide synthesis inhibitor	• Second-line drug for TB treatment • Treatment of multidrug-resistant TB	• Ototoxicity • Nephrotoxicity • Local injection site reactions
Cycloserine (Seromycin)	• **A:** PO • **E:** Majority excreted unchanged in urine	**MOA:** • Cell wall synthesis inhibitor	• Second-line drug for TB treatment	• Side effects limit clinical usefulness • Peripheral neuropathy • CNS dysfunction (depression and psychosis) • Pyridoxine coadministration can reduce CNS side effects

Ciprofloxacin (Cipro) and Levofloxacin (Levaquin)	• **A:** PO (well absorbed) and IV • **D:** Widely distributed to most tissues • **M:** Hepatic metabolism • **E:** Parent drug and metabolites excreted in urine and feces	**MOA:** • Block bacterial DNA synthesis by inhibiting DNA gyrase **Resistance:** • Via mutations in DNA gyrase	• Primary indication in multidrug combination for *M avium intracellulare* complex in late stage AIDS • Second-line in multidrug combination to treat TB resistant to first-line drugs	• Minimal
Ethionamide (Trecator-SC)	• **A:** PO • **D:** Crosses BBB • **M:** Hepatic metabolism • **E:** Parent drug and metabolites excreted in urine	**MOA:** • Similar structure to isoniazid • Inhibits the synthesis of mycolic acids • Mycolic acids are essential components of the mycobacterial cell wall	• Second-line drug for TB treatment	• Side effects limit clinical usefulness • Intense gastric irritation • Adverse neurologic effects • Hepatotoxic • Pyridoxine coadministration can reduce CNS side effects
p-Aminosalicyclic Acid/ PAS (Paser)	• **A:** PO; readily absorbed • **D:** Widely distributed; does not cross BBB • **E:** Parent drug and metabolites excreted in urine	**MOA:** • Inhibits folic acid synthesis	• Second-line drug for TB treatment	• GI irritation • Crystalluria • Peptic ulceration • Hypersensitivity reactions (fever, rash, hepatitis, granulocytopenia) • Primary resistance is common • Resistance limits usefulness

Continued

ANTIMYCOBACTERIALS: DRUG FACTS (Continued)

Drug	Pharmacokinetics	Mechanisms of Action and of Resistance	Clinical Uses and General Information	Drawbacks and Side Effects
Rifabutin (Mycobutin)	• **A:** PO • **M:** Metabolized by hepatic P450 enzymes • **E:** Metabolites excreted in urine and feces	**MOA:** • Inhibits RNA synthesis by binding to the β subunit of DNA-dependent RNA polymerase in susceptible microorganisms • Inhibits protein synthesis by preventing chain initiation • Virtually no effect on mammalian RNA polymerase • Tuberculocidal to intracellular and extracellular organisms	• Second-line drug for TB treatment • Prevention and treatment of atypical mycobacterial infection in AIDS patients with CD4 counts below 50 μL	• Drug interactions due to induction of P450 enzymes
Dapsone	• **A:** PO; well absorbed • **D:** Widely distributed • **M:** Hepatic metabolism • **E:** Unchanged and acetylated compound excreted in urine	**MOA:** • Inhibits folic acid synthesis	• Treatment of leprosy • Treatment and prophylaxis of PCP in AIDS patients	• GI irritation • Fever • Skin rashes • Methemoglobinemia • Hemolysis (especially in patients with G6PD deficiency)
Clofazimine (Lamprene)	• **A:** PO; variable absorption • **E:** In feces	**MOA:** • Unknown • May involve DNA binding	• Treatment of dapsone-resistant leprosy	• Skin discoloration • GI irritation

CHAPTER 3

AUTONOMIC NERVOUS SYSTEM STRUCTURE AND MEDICATIONS

I. STRUCTURE

ANS Components

Overview of ANS and Actions of Some Drugs

Effects of ANS on Organ Systems

II. MEDICATIONS

Classification of Cholinergic Agonists

Direct Cholinergic Agonists: Acetylcholine Agonists

Indirect Cholinergic Agonists: Antiacetylcholinesterases

Classification of Muscarinic Antagonists

Muscarinic Antagonists

Classification of Ganglionic Blockers

Ganglionic Blockers

Classification of Sympathomimetics

Catecholamines

Noncatecholamines

Effects of Sympathomimetics on Organ Systems

Classification of Adrenergic Blockers

α-Blockers and Neuronal Blockers

β-Blockers

III. PHARMACOLOGY OF THE EYE

Cholinergic and Adrenergic Drugs for Treating Conditions of the Eye

Eye Receptor Mechanisms

Medications for Treating Diseases of the Eye

Clinically Important Structures of the Eye and Their Receptors

TERMS TO LEARN

Acetylcholinesterase	Enzyme responsible for the degradation of Ach.
Adrenergic Neuronal Blockers	Medications that prevent NE from exiting the nerve terminal.
Anisocoria	Unequal pupils.
Intrinsic Sympathomimetic Activity (ISA)	Drugs with paradoxical partial β-agonist properties; clinical significance unknown.
Lipid Solubility	Accounts for the CNS side effects of a drug.
Malignant Hypertension	Severely elevated blood pressure associated with CNS, renal, or cardiac symptoms.
Membrane Stabilizing Activity (MSA)	Imparts a local anesthetic quality to β-blockers; may contribute to antiarrhythmic property.
Miosis	Pupillary constriction.
Myasthenia Gravis	Autoimmune disease characterized by increasing muscle weakness with use due to the presence of antibodies to the Ach receptor at the neuromuscular junction.
Mydriasis	Pupillary dilation.
Nonselective α-Adrenergic Blockers	Medications that block α_1- and α_2-adrenergic sites.
Nonselective β-Blockers	Medications that block β_1- and β_2-adrenergic sites.
Pheochromocytoma	Tumor of the adrenal gland that secretes catecholamines. (NE,D,Epi)
Plasma Binding	Accounts for the drug interactions.
Postural (orthostatic) Hypotension	A 20 mm Hg drop in systolic blood pressure or 10 mm Hg drop in diastolic blood pressure within 3 minutes of standing due to a defect in the blood pressure control system.
Raynaud's Disease	Vascular disorder characterized by peripheral vasoconstriction.

Selective α-Adrenergic Blockers	Medications that block α_1-adrenergic sites only.
Selective β-Adrenergic Blockers	Medications that block β_1-adrenergic sites only.
Sjögren's Syndrome	Syndrome of dry mouth and dry eyes due to lymphocytic infiltration of the salivary and lacrimal glands; often observed in patients with autoimmune disorders including RA and SLE.
Tourette's Syndrome	Syndrome characterized by motor and verbal tics.
Xerostomia	Dry mouth.

I. Structure

ANS COMPONENTS

Component	Parasympathetic Nervous System	Sympathetic Nervous System
Path of preganglionic cell	CN III, VII, IX, X, and S2–S4	TI–L2
Preganglionic fiber length	Long	Short
Preganglionic myelination	Myelinated	Myelinated
Pre- to postganglionic ratio	One to one (except vagus nerve)	One to many
Preganglionic cell NT	Ach	Ach
Postganglionic cell location	On or near organ	Sympathetic chain next to spinal cord
Postganglionic fiber length	Short	Long
Postganglionic myelination	Unmyelinated	Unmyelinated
Postganglionic cell NT	Ach	NE (except adrenal medulla—EPI; piloerector muscles and sweat glands—Ach)

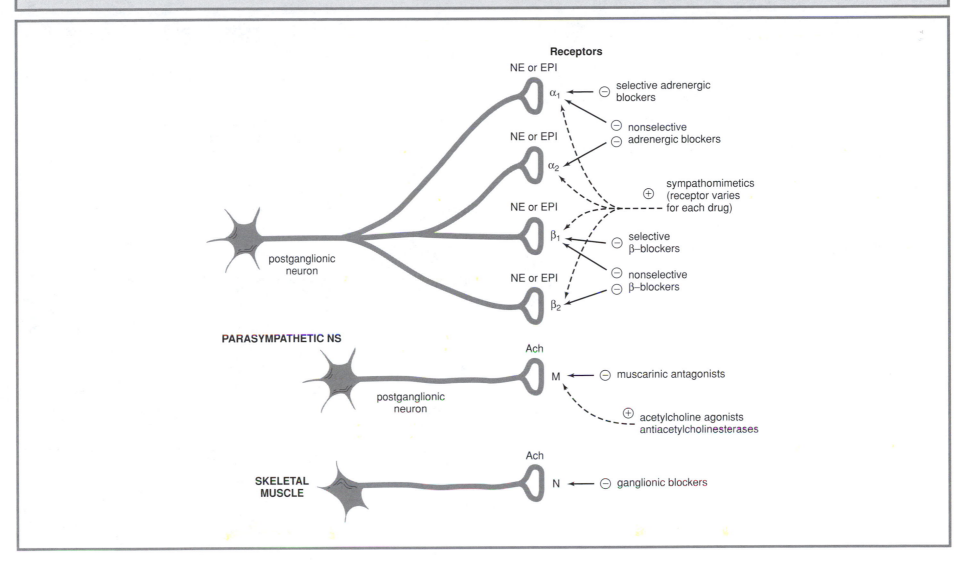

EFFECTS OF ANS ON ORGAN SYSTEMS

Tissue	Parasympathetic Nervous System		Sympathetic Nervous System	
	Mechanism	Effect	Mechanism	Effect
Pupil of the eye α_1 M	• Ach binds to muscarinic receptors on the sphincter muscle • Ach binds to muscarinic receptor on the ciliary muscle (Note: Contraction of ciliary muscle causes relaxation of the suspensory ligaments, allowing the lens to get rounder and facilitates near vision)	• Contraction of the sphincter muscle leads to constriction of the pupil • Contraction of ciliary muscle (causes opening of canal of Schlemm, which leads to decreased intraocular pressure)	NE or EPI binds to α_1-receptors on the radial muscles	Contraction of the radial muscles leads to dilation of the pupil
Bronchi α_1 β_2 M	Ach binds to muscarinic receptors	Contracts smooth muscle surrounding bronchi	• NE or EPI binds to α_1-receptors • NE or EPI binds to β_2-receptors	Increases organic content of secretions Relaxation of smooth muscles surrounding bronchi
Heart β_1 M	Ach binds to muscarinic receptors	Decrease in heart rate and ionotropy	NE or EPI binds to β_1-receptors	Increase in heart rate and ionotropy
Blood vessels α_1 β_2 M	Ach from exogenous source (no direct parasympathetic innervation of the blood vessels)	Vasodilation	• NE or EPI binds to α_1-receptors on all blood vessels except those supplying skeletal muscles • NE or EPI binds to β_2-receptors on blood vessels that supply skeletal muscles	• Vasoconstriction • Vasodilation
GI tract M β_2	• Ach binds to muscarinic receptors on longitudinal muscles	• Contraction of longitudinal muscles	• NE or EPI on β_2-receptors on longitudinal muscles	• Relaxation of longitudinal muscles

α_1 M *(handwritten)*	• Ach binds to muscarinic receptors on sphincter muscles	• Relaxation of sphincter muscles • Both lead to increased peristalsis and bowel movements	• NE or EPI binds to α_1-receptors on sphincter muscles	• Contraction of sphincter muscles • Both effects result in decrease of bowel movement
Bladder $\beta_2 \alpha_1$ M *(handwritten)*	• Ach binds to muscarinic receptors on body of bladder • Ach binds to muscarinic receptors on sphincter of the bladder	• Contraction of body of bladder • Relaxation of the sphincter of the bladder • Both effects result in urination	• NE or EPI binds to β_2-receptors on the body of the bladder • NE or EPI binds to α_1-receptors on the sphincter of the bladder	• Relaxation of the body of the bladder • Contraction of the sphincter of the bladder • Both effects result in decreased urination
Liver β_2 *(handwritten)*	Impulses via vagus nerve	Slight glycogen synthesis; weak gallbladder contraction	NE or EPI binds to β_2-receptors	Increase in glycogenolysis and gluconeogenesis
Pancreas $\beta_2 \alpha_2$ *(handwritten)*	Impulses via vagus nerve Ach release	Secretion of moderate to large amounts of enzymes into the pancreatic acini	• NE or EPI binds to β_2-receptors on the beta cells • NE or EPI binds to α_2-receptors on the beta cells	• Increase in insulin release (predominant effect) • Decrease in insulin release
Kidney	Insignificant	Insignificant	NE or EPI binds to β_1-receptors	Renin release
Adipose tissue	Insignificant	Insignificant	NE binds to β_3-receptors on adipocytes	Increased lipolysis (release of free fatty acids)

II. Medications

CLASSIFICATION OF CHOLINERGIC AGONISTS

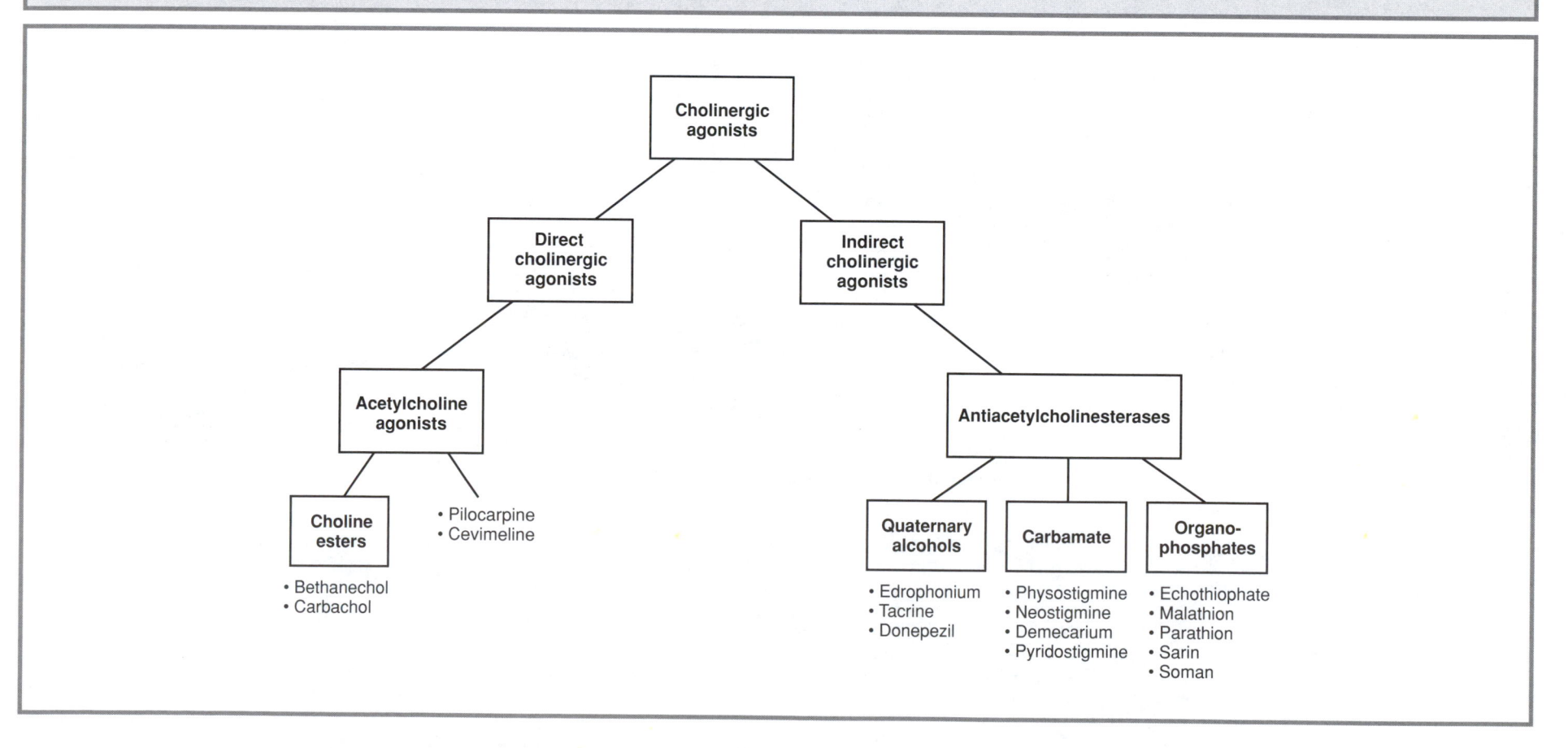

DIRECT CHOLINERGIC AGONISTS: ACETYLCHOLINE AGONISTS

Drug	Pharmacokinetics	Mechanism of Action	Clinical Uses	Drawbacks and Side Effects
Bethanechol (Urecholine, Duvoid, Urabeth)	• **A:** PO and SC • **D:** Poor lipid solubility; does not cross the BBB • **DOA:** Longer duration of action than acetylcholine due to resistance to cholinesterases	• Favors M receptors (especially M_3)	• Enhance normal functioning of GI tract and bladder postoperatively	**Contraindications:** • Asthma—increase bronchial constriction and secretions • Hyperthyroidism • Coronary insufficiency—stimulation of M receptors in coronary arteries causes vasoconstriction • Peptic ulcer disease
Carbachol (Isopto Carbachol, Miostat, Carboptic)	• **A:** Ophthalmic drops and intraoptic • **D:** Poor lipid solubility; does not cross the BBB • **DOA:** Longer duration of action than acetylcholine due to resistance to acetylcholinesterase	• More N than M activity	• Wide-angle glaucoma (acts by constricting the ciliary muscle, which opens the meshwork of the canal of Schlemm)	**Muscarinic Poisoning Symptoms = Parasympathetic Overdrive** • Salivation and lacrimation • Nausea and vomiting
Pilocarpine (Isopto Carpine, Salagen)	• **A:** PO and ophthalmic drops; well absorbed • **D:** Good lipid solubility	• Favors M receptors	• Wide-angle glaucoma (acts by constricting the ciliary muscle, which opens the meshwork of the canal of Schlemm) • Used to treat xerostomia in patients with head and neck cancers	• Headache and visual disturbances • Bronchospasm • Bradycardia and hypotension
Cevimeline (Evoxac)	• **A:** PO • **D:** Moderate lipid solubility • **M:** Hepatic metabolism by P450 enzymes • **E:** Parent drug and metabolites excreted in urine	• Favors M receptors	• Treatment of xerostomia associated with Sjögren's syndrome	• Shock • Diarrhea • Urination **These symptoms can be reversed with administration of atropine**

INDIRECT CHOLINERGIC AGONISTS: ANTIACETYLCHOLINESTERASES

Drug	Pharmacokinetics	Mechanism of Action	Clinical Uses	Drawbacks and Side Effects
Quaternary Alcohols				
Edrophonium (Enlon, Tensilon)	• **A:** IM and IV • **D:** No CNS effects • **E:** In urine	• Reversibly bind directly to acetylcholinesterase	• Diagnosis of myasthenia gravis	**Poisoning symptoms:** ☞ **DUMBELS** • Diarrhea • Urination • Miosis • Bronchoconstriction • Excitation (skeletal muscle and CNS) • Lacrimation • Salivation and sweating • Poisoning can be treated with atropine • Use of tacrine is limited due to hepatotoxicity
Tacrine (Cognex) 10, 20, 30, 40 mg caps QID dosing	• **A:** PO • **D:** Enters the CNS • **M:** Metabolized by hepatic P450 enzymes • **E:** Not fully elucidated; small amounts excreted in urine		• Treatment of Alzheimer's disease	
Donepezil (Aricept) 5, 10 mg tab qdaily	• **A:** PO • **M:** Metabolized by hepatic P450 enzymes • **E:** Parent drug and metabolites excreted in urine			
Carbamates				
Physostigmine (Isopto Eserine, Antilirium)	• **A:** IM, IV, and ophthalmic • **M:** Hydrolyzed by cholinesterases, degraded more slowly than Ach • **E:** Not fully elucidated; small amounts excreted in urine	• Reversibly bind directly to acetylcholinesterase	• Applied topically for wide-angle glaucoma • Treatment of CNS toxicity associated with anticholinergic poisoning	Same as above.

Neostigmine (Prostigmin)	• **A:** IM, IV, SC, and PO • **M:** Hydrolyzed by cholinesterases • **E:** Parent drug and metabolites excreted in urine		• Drug of choice for paralytic ileus and atony of the bladder from surgery • Treatment and diagnosis of myasthenia gravis • Reversal of NM blockade	
Pyridostigmine (Mestinon)	• **A:** IM, IV, and PO • **M:** Hydrolyzed by cholinesterases • **E:** Majority excreted unchanged in urine		• Treatment of myasthenia gravis • Pretreatment to reduce risk of mortality on exposure to "nerve gases" • Reversal of NM blockade	
Demecarium (Humorsol)	• **A:** Ophthalmic		• Glaucoma	
Organophosphates				
Echothiophate (Phospholine iodide) Malathion (Ovide) Parathion Sarin and Soman	• **A:** Well absorbed through skin, lung, gut, and conjunctiva • **M:** Metabolized (especially in insects) by mixed function oxygenases to active form (ie, parathion to paraxin and malathion to malaoxon)	• Irreversibly bind to acetylcholinesterase (exception: malathion, which binds reversibly and is the least toxic of the class)	• Glaucoma (second-line agent) • Treatment of head lice • Used in insecticides • Nerve gases (highly volatile liquids that are among the most toxic synthetic agents known) • Sarin was used in terrorist attack in Japanese subway	• Poisoning symptoms as above • Poisoning (aside from CNS symptoms) can be treated with atropine • Poisoning can be reversed with pralidoxime (2-PAM) • Parathion causes most cases of poisoning and death associated with organophosphates

CLASSIFICATION OF MUSCARINIC ANTAGONISTS

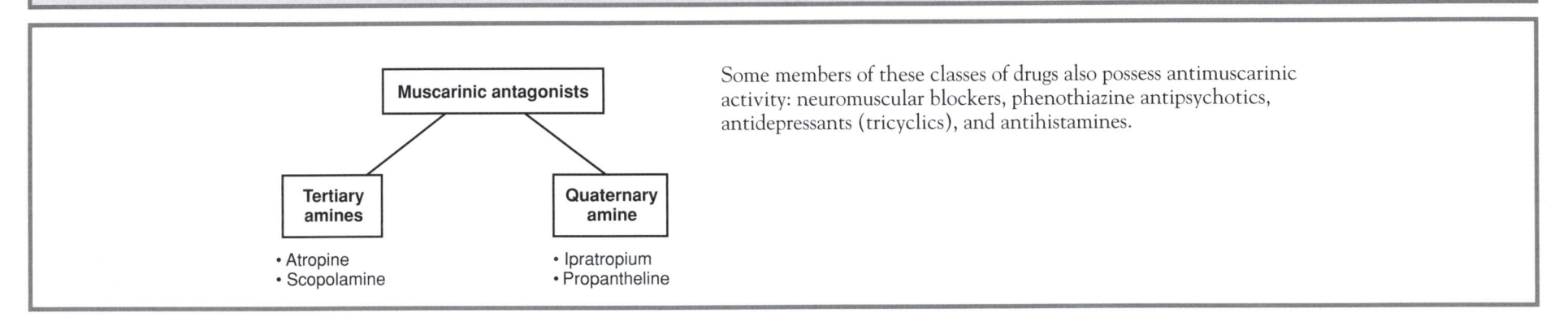

Some members of these classes of drugs also possess antimuscarinic activity: neuromuscular blockers, phenothiazine antipsychotics, antidepressants (tricyclics), and antihistamines.

MUSCARINIC ANTAGONISTS

Drug	Pharmacokinetics	Mechanism of Action	Clinical Uses	Drawbacks and Side Effects	Toxicity of Muscarinic Antagonists
Tertiary Amines					
Atropine (Sal-Tropine, Isopto Atropine)	• **A:** Endotracheal, IM, IV, PO, SC, and ophthalmic drops • **D:** Well distributed; crosses BBB • **M:** Hepatic metabolism • **E:** Parent drug and metabolites excreted in urine	• Act as competitive inhibitors • Effects can be overcome by increased concentrations of muscarinic agonists	• Reverse muscarinic or antiacetylcholine sterase poisoning • Mydriasis with cycloplegia • Mydriasis for prolonged periods of time • Cardiac arrest	**Contraindications:** • Can precipitate acute glaucoma in patients with narrow anterior chamber angle • Can precipitate hyperthermia in infants • Should not be used in men with BPH	☞ • Mouth (dry) • Urinary retention • Skin (hot and flushed) • Constipation • Airway dilation and reduction of secretions • Rhythm disturbance (tachycardia) • Intraventricular conduction may be blocked • Nervous system (CNS confusion) • Eyes (mydriasis) OR Adage "dry as a bone, blind as a bat, red as a beet, mad as a hatter"
Scopolamine (Isopto Hyoscine, Hyoscine) _5,15mL_ _(handwritten)_ _Transderm Scop 1.5mg patch_ _(handwritten)_	• **A:** IM, IV, PO, SC, ophthalmic, or transdermal patch • **D:** Crosses BBB • **M:** Hepatic metabolism • **E:** Metabolites excreted in urine		• Treatment and prevention of motion sickness • Ophthalmologic applications (see Medications for Treating Diseases of the Eye)		

Continued

MUSCARINIC ANTAGONISTS (Continued)

Drug	Pharmacokinetics	Mechanism of Action	Clinical Uses	Drawbacks and Side Effects	Toxicity of Muscarinic Antagonists
Quaternary Amines					
Ipratropium (Atrovent) *nasal spray 0.03% 2 spays 2-3×day inhalation 2 inh QID*	• **A:** Inhaled • **D:** Poorly absorbed; does not cross BBB • **E:** In urine and feces		• Bronchodilator in asthma and COPD	• Less risk of side effects due to poor distribution • Can precipitate hyperthermia in infants • Should not be used in men with BPH	
Propantheline (Pro-Banthine)	• **A:** PO • **D:** Poorly absorbed; does not cross BBB • **M:** In GI tract and liver • **E:** Parent drug and metabolites excreted in urine		• Decrease acid secretion in patients with PUD		

Trevor AJ, Katzung BG, Masters SB: *Katzung & Trevor's Pharmacology Examination & Board Review*. 6th ed. McGraw-Hill; 2002.

CLASSIFICATION OF GANGLIONIC BLOCKERS

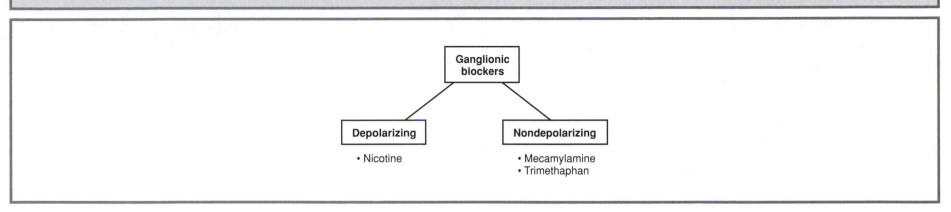

3. Autonomic Nervous System Structure and Medications

GANGLIONIC BLOCKERS

Drug	Pharmacokinetics	Mechanism of Action	Clinical Uses	Drawbacks and Side Effects
Nicotine (Nicoderm, Nicotrol, Nicotrol inhaler, Nicorette)	• **A:** Inhaler, nasal spray, buccal, or transdermal • **M:** Liver, kidney, and lungs • **E:** Parent drug and metabolites excreted in urine	• Blockade via persistent depolarization • Stimulation of autonomic ganglia (parasympathetic and sympathetic) followed by blockade • Stimulation of adrenal medulla • Stimulation of CNS (alerting response, change in respiration)	• Treatment of nicotine addiction	**Mild:** • Vomiting • Transient increase in salivation • Cold sweat • Disturbed vision • Dizziness • Muscular weakness **Severe:** • Tachycardia and arrhythmia • Respiratory distress • Convulsion • Death
Mecamylamine (Inversine)	• **A:** PO • **E:** Unchanged in urine	• Competitive pharmacologic antagonists • Block both parasympathetic and sympathetic systems • These drugs were the first used to treat hypertension; however, their use for this condition is limited due to excessive side effects	• Treatment of moderate to severe hypertension • Treatment of uncomplicated malignant hypertension • Possible use in Tourette's syndrome and nicotine addiction	• Extensive side effects have led to limited clinical usefulness of nondepolarizing ganglionic blockers • Postural hypotension • Xerostomia • Blurred vision • Constipation • Severe sexual dysfunction
Trimethaphan (Arfonad)	• **A:** IV • **E:** Majority excreted unchanged in urine		• Treatment of malignant hypertension	

CLASSIFICATION OF SYMPATHOMIMETICS

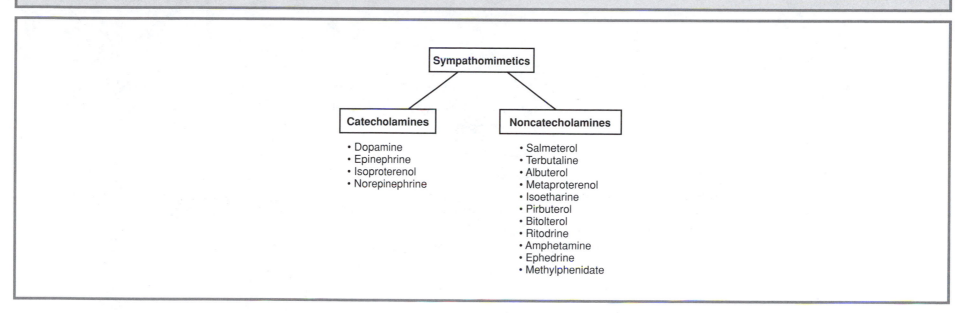

Sympathomimetics

Catecholamines

- Dopamine
- Epinephrine
- Isoproterenol
- Norepinephrine

Noncatecholamines

- Salmeterol
- Terbutaline
- Albuterol
- Metaproterenol
- Isoetharine
- Pirbuterol
- Bitolterol
- Ritodrine
- Amphetamine
- Ephedrine
- Methylphenidate

CATECHOLAMINES

Drug	Pharmacokinetics	Mechanism of Action	Clinical Uses	Drawbacks and Side Effects
Dopamine (Intropin)	• A: IV	• Stimulates NE release • α_1-, α_2-, and β_1-Agonist	• Treatment of cardiogenic shock • Treatment of CHF • Treatment of acute renal failure • Important for its ability to maintain renal blood flow	• High doses can lead to vasoconstriction through α stimulation
Epinephrine (Adrenaline, Epipen, Epifrin)	• A: IV, IM, PO, SC, intracardiac, endotracheal, and topical	• α_1-, α_2-, β_1-, and β_2-Agonist	• Lowering intraocular pressure in wide-angle glaucoma • Combined with local anesthetics to prolong their action • Topical use for hemostasis • Treatment of complete heart block or cardiac arrest • Bronchodilator for treatment of asthma • Treatment of anaphylactic shock	• HR increases • BP increases (pulse pressure increases) • TPR decreases slightly
Isoproterenol (Isuprel)	• A: IM, IV, SC, and inhaled	• β_1- and β_2-Agonist	• Bronchodilator for treatment of asthma • Complete heart block or cardiac arrest • Shock	• HR increases • BP decreases (pulse pressure increases) • TPR decreases
Norepinephrine (Levophed)	• A: IV	• α_1- and α_2-Agonist • Some β_1 activation	• Treatment of hypotension (causes vasoconstriction)	• HR decreases (vagal-mediated central reflex) • BP increases (pulse pressure same) • TPR increases

NONCATECHOLAMINES

Drug	Pharmacokinetics	Mechanism of Action	Clinical Uses	Drawbacks and Side Effects
Salmeterol (Serevent)	• A: Inhaled	• β_2-Agonists	• Bronchodilators for treatment of asthma	• Minimal side effects
Terbutaline (Brethine)	• A: Inhaled, PO, and SC		• Salmeterol is best choice for prophylaxis because it is a longer acting bronchodilator	• Skeletal muscle tremor
Albuterol (Proventil, Ventolin)	• A: Inhaled and PO		• Terbutaline and Ritodrine also used to stop premature contractions in pregnant women	
Metaproterenol (Metaprel, Alupent)				
Isoetharine	• A: Inhaled			
Pirbuterol (Maxair)				
Bitolterol (Tornolate)				
Ritodrine	• A: IV and PO			
Amphetamine (Adderall)	• A: PO	• α- and β-Agonist • Causes release of DA, NE, and 5-HT from nerve terminal	• Treatment of ADHD • Treatment of narcolepsy • Treatment of exogenous obesity	• Restlessness • Tremor • Insomnia • Anxiety • Tachycardia
Ephedrine	• A: IM, IV, PO, and SC	• α- and β-Agonist • Causes release of NE	• Bronchodilator for treatment of asthma • Treatment of nasal congestion • Treatment of hypotension and shock	
Methylphenidate (Ritalin)	• A: PO	• Blocks reuptake of NE	• Treatment of ADHD • Treatment of narcolepsy	

EFFECTS OF SYMPATHOMIMETICS ON ORGAN SYSTEMS

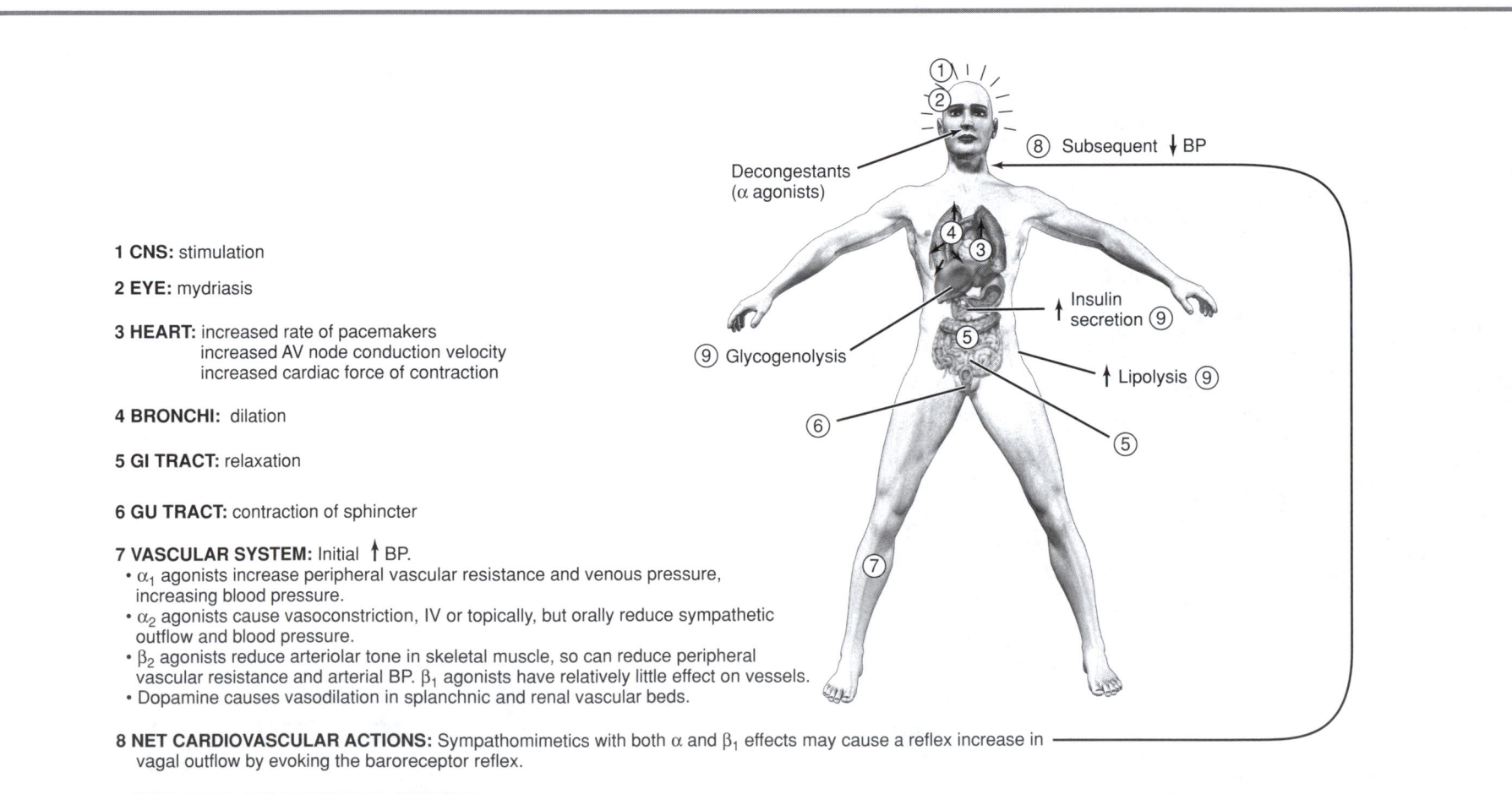

1 CNS: stimulation

2 EYE: mydriasis

3 HEART: increased rate of pacemakers
increased AV node conduction velocity
increased cardiac force of contraction

4 BRONCHI: dilation

5 GI TRACT: relaxation

6 GU TRACT: contraction of sphincter

7 VASCULAR SYSTEM: Initial ↑ BP.
- α_1 agonists increase peripheral vascular resistance and venous pressure, increasing blood pressure.
- α_2 agonists cause vasoconstriction, IV or topically, but orally reduce sympathetic outflow and blood pressure.
- β_2 agonists reduce arteriolar tone in skeletal muscle, so can reduce peripheral vascular resistance and arterial BP. β_1 agonists have relatively little effect on vessels.
- Dopamine causes vasodilation in splanchnic and renal vascular beds.

8 NET CARDIOVASCULAR ACTIONS: Sympathomimetics with both α and β_1 effects may cause a reflex increase in vagal outflow by evoking the baroreceptor reflex.

9 METABOLIC AND HORMONAL EFFECTS:
- β_1 agonists increase renin secretion.
- β_2 agonists increase insulin secretion by the pancreas and glycogenolysis in the liver.
- All β agonists appear to stimulate lipolysis.

Image labels:
Decongestants (α agonists)
⑧ Subsequent ↓ BP
↑ Insulin secretion ⑨
⑨ Glycogenolysis
↑ Lipolysis ⑨

CLASSIFICATION OF ADRENERGIC BLOCKERS

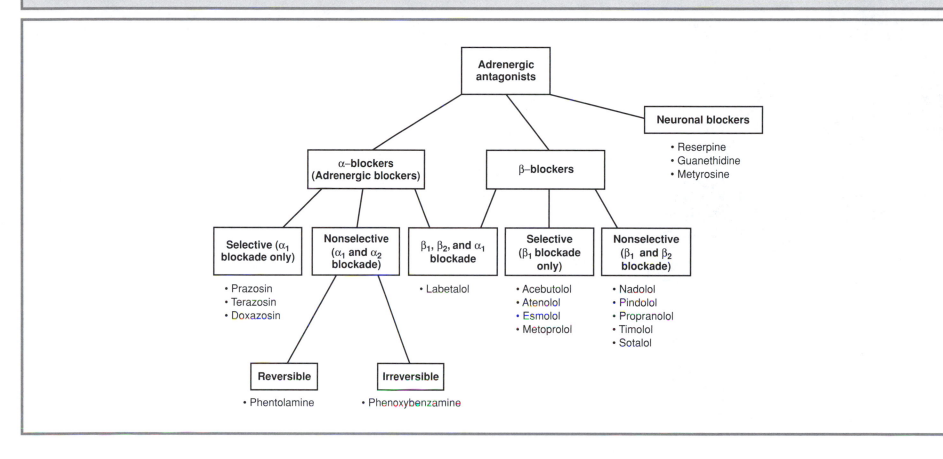

α-BLOCKERS AND NEURONAL BLOCKERS

Drug	Pharmacokinetics	Mechanism of Action	Clinical Uses	Drawbacks and Side Effects
Nonselective α-Adrenergic Blocker (Reversible)				
Phentolamine (Regitine)	• **A:** IV or IM • **E:** Some excreted unchanged in urine	• Decreases in TPR and BP through action upon α-receptors in vascular smooth muscle • Orthostatic hypotension via antagonism of sympathetic stimulation of α_1-receptors in venous smooth muscle • Big increase in HR due to decreased autoregulation by α_2-receptor blocking	• Once used to diagnose pheochromocytoma • Blocks vasoconstriction to increase tissue perfusion in patients with shock • Treatment of hypertensive emergencies • Peripheral vasodilation in conditions such as Raynaud's disease • Treatment of erectile dysfunction	• Severe tachycardia • Arrhythmias • Myocardial ischemia • Orthostatic hypotension • Diarrhea • Increased gastric acid production
Nonselective α-Adrenergic Blocker (Irreversible)				
Phenoxybenzamine (Dibenzyline)	• **A:** PO • **DOA:** Long (3–4 days) • **M:** Hepatic metabolites • **E:** Metabolites excreted in urine and feces	• Blocks catecholamine induced vasoconstriction • Increased CO due to reflex tachycardia • Prevention of symptoms of pheochromocytoma via α blockade	• Diagnosis and treatment of pheochromocytoma • Peripheral vasodilation in conditions such as Raynaud's disease	• Enters CNS causing sedation and fatigue • Orthostatic hypotension

Selective α_1-Adrenergic Blockers

Prazosin (Minipress) Terazosin (Hytrin) Doxazosin (Cardura)	• **A:** PO • **M:** Hepatic metabolism • **E:** Majority of parent drug and metabolites excreted in feces; remainder in urine	• Relaxation of arterial and venous smooth muscle via α_1 blockade	• Treatment of BPH • Treatment of hypertension	• Exaggerated orthostatic hypotension response to first dose in some patients so should be taken at bedtime

Neuronal Blockers

Reserpine (Serpasil)	• **A:** PO • **M:** Hepatic metabolism to inactive metabolites • **E:** Metabolites excreted in urine and feces	• Blocks reuptake of NE, DA, and 5-HT into vesicle • Results in depletion of DA, NE, and 5-HT from central and peripheral neurons	• Treatment of mild to moderate hypertension	• Diarrhea • Parkinson-like syndrome • Sedation • Severe depression and suicide
Guanethidine (Ismelin)	• **A:** PO • **M:** Hepatic metabolism • **E:** Parent drug and metabolites in urine	• Replaces NE bound to ATP in vesicles • Prevents NE release from peripheral nerve terminals	• Treatment of hypertension	• Rarely used due to side effects • Orthostatic hypotension • Severe diarrhea • Sexual dysfunction
Metyrosine (Demser)	• **A:** PO • **E:** Majority excreted unchanged in urine	• Blocks tyrosine hydroxylase • Interferes with DA synthesis • Therefore, there is less NE and EPI secreted by the tumor	• Treatment of pheochromocytoma (especially in patients with metastatic or inoperable disease)	• Crystalluria • Sedation • Diarrhea • Anxiety

β-BLOCKERS

Drug	Pharmacokinetics							Mechanisms of Clinical Effects	Clinical Uses	Drawbacks and Side Effects
	Selective	Lipid Solubility	Plasma Binding	$t_{1/2}$ (hours)	Route	ISA	MSA			
Acebutolol (Sectral)	Yes, affinity for β_1 sites only	Low	Low	3–4	PO	Yes	Yes	• Treatment of hypertension via decreased HR, CO, contractility, renin release by kidney, and BP via CNS actions • Treatment of angina via decreased HR, contractility, heart work, and oxygen consumption • Treatment of hyperthyroidism by blocking thyroxin, which causes β_1 stimulation of the heart	• Hypertension • Angina • Hyperthyroidism	**Contraindications:** • Acute CHF (except pindolol) • Asthma (use selective β-blockers) **Side Effects:** • CNS—insomnia, sedation (especially with Propranolol) • CVS—bradycardia and hypotension (selectives and nonselectives) • Cold extremities (nonselectives only) • Bronchoconstriction therefore use selective blockers cautiously
Atenolol (Tenormin)	Yes, β_1 affinity	Low	Low	6–9	PO, IV	No	No		• Hypertension • Angina • Hyperthyroidism	
Esmolol (Brevibloc)	Yes, β_1 affinity	Low	Low	10 min	IV	No	No		• Arrhythmias	
Metoprolol (Toprol, Lopressor)	Yes, β_1 affinity	Moderate	Low	3–4	PO, IV	No	Yes		• Hypertension • Angina • Hyperthyroidism	
Nadolol (Corgard)	No, affinity for β_1 and β_2 sites	Low	Low	24	PO	No	No			
Pindolol (Viskin)		Moderate		3–4	PO	Yes (high)	Yes			

Propranolol (Inderal)	☞ **Non**selective **Nadolol Pin**ned **Tim's Prop** on **Sota**	High	High, >90%	3–6	PO, IV	No	Yes, high	• Treats glaucoma by decreasing production of aqueous humor	• Arrhythmias • Hypertension • Angina • Hyperthyroidism • Migraine • Situational phobias
Timolol (Blocadren, Timoptic)	No, β_1 and β_2 affinity	Moderate	Low	4–5	PO, ophthalmic	No	No		• Glaucoma • Hypertension • Angina • Hyperthyroidism
Sotalol (Betapace)	No, β_1 and β_2 affinity	Low	Low	3–6	PO	No	No		• Hypertension • Angina • Hyperthyroidism
Labetalol (Normodyne, Trandate)	No (affinity for β_1, β_2, and α_1 sites)	Moderate	Low	3–6	PO and IV	No	Yes		• Hypertension

III. Pharmacology of the Eye

CHOLINERGIC AND ADRENERGIC DRUGS FOR TREATING CONDITIONS OF THE EYE

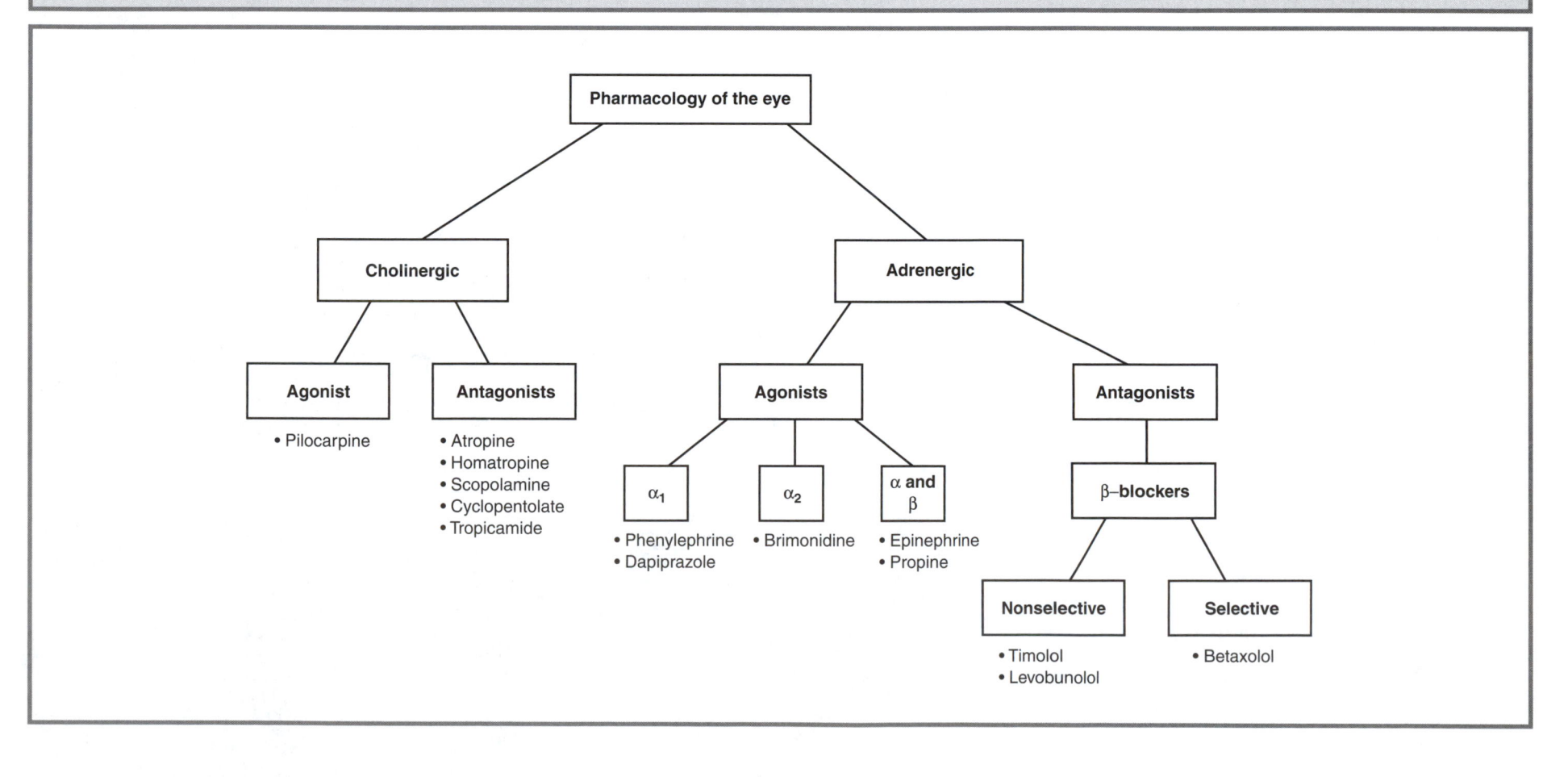

EYE RECEPTOR MECHANISMS

Area	Mechanism
Dilator muscle	• Adrenergic stimulation of α_1-receptors on muscle causes pupil to dilate.
Pupillary sphincter muscles	• Cholinergic stimulation of muscarinic receptors on these muscles cause the pupils to constrict.
Ciliary body	• Cholinergic stimulation of muscarinic receptors causes a contraction of the ciliary body leading to increased accommodation. • Adrenergic stimulation causes ciliary muscle to relax, allowing for far vision; produces aqueous humor.

MEDICATIONS FOR TREATING DISEASES OF THE EYE

Drug	Mechanism of Action	Clinical Uses	Drawbacks and Side Effects*
Pilocarpine (Pilagan)	• Causes miosis via constriction of the pupillary sphincter muscle • Increases accommodation via constriction of the ciliary muscle • Reduces intraocular pressure by widening trabecular spaces to increase outflow of aqueous humor	• Testing for anisocoria (will not constrict a pharmacologically dilated pupil) • Treatment of glaucoma	• Nearsightedness • Decreased vision (problem in people with cataracts)
Atropine (Isopto Atropine) Homatropine (Isopto Homatropine) Scopolamine (Isopto Hyoscine)	• Cholinergic antagonist at muscarinic receptors on the iris and ciliary body causes cycloplegia and mydriasis • Long acting (hours to days) ☞ Cholinergic Antagonists Have Systemic Toxicity	• Decrease post surgical inflammation (prevents iris from adhering to the cornea and relaxes the ciliary muscle and reduces vascular permeability) • Prevent adhesion formation in iritis, uveitis, and postoperatively • Dilation for eye examinations	• May precipitate acute glaucoma in patients with a narrow anterior chamber angle • Risk of antimuscarinic poisoning if enters systemic circulation

*Eye drops must be used with care because they can cause lethal complications, such as hypertensive crisis and ventricular arrhythmias.

Continued

MEDICATIONS FOR TREATING DISEASES OF THE EYE (Continued)

Drug	Mechanism of Action	Clinical Uses	Drawbacks and Side Effects*
Cyclopentolate (Cyclogyl)	See page 101.	• Good for corneal abrasions (decreases pain from ciliary muscle spasm) or mild conditions where cycloplegia and mydriasis are desired	• Risk of antimuscarinic poisoning if enters systemic circulation
Tropicamide (Mydriacyl)		• Produces dilation of pupil; useful for funduscopic examinations	• Blurred vision • Headache • Sensitivity to light • Risk of antimuscarinic poisoning if enters systemic circulation
Phenylephrine (Neosynephrine)	• α_1-Agonist at radial muscle of the iris	• Often added in small concentration to OTC drops to whiten the sclera via vasoconstriction	• Causes rebound dilation and redder eyes
Dapiprazole (Rev Eyes)		• Helps reverse the effects of iatrogenic dilation following an eye examination	• Conjunctival irritation
Brimonidine (Alphagan)	• Reduces production of aqueous humor • Increases outflow of aqueous humor	• Treatment of glaucoma • Treatment of ocular hypertension	• Burning, stinging of the eye • Blurred vision
Epinephrine (Epifrin, Glaucon)	• Causes conjunctival constriction • Causes slight mydriasis • Reduces intraocular pressure (mainly by increasing outflow and slight decrease in aqueous humor production)	• Treatment of glaucoma by reducing intraocular pressure via increased outflow and decreased production of aqueous humor	• Localized burning and irritation • Localized allergic reaction • Accumulation of melanin granules • Can cause lethal hypertensive crisis or ventricular arrhythmias by entering systemic vasculature via nasal cavity from tear duct
Propine (Dipivefrin)	• Transformed into epinephrine once in the eye and has same beneficial effects	• Treatment of glaucoma • Lipophilic version of epinephrine (leads to better absorption through the cornea)	• Absorption into the eye reduces therapeutic dose so systemic side effects of epinephrine are decreased

Timolol (Timoptic)	• Theoretically decreases aqueous humor formation via receptors on the ciliary body	• Drug of choice for glaucoma	• Localized irritation and burning
Levobunolol (Betagan)		• Treatment of glaucoma • Less expensive than timolol	• CNS effects include lethargy, light-headedness, fatigue, memory loss • CV effects include bradycardia, hypotension, syncope, arrhythmias, wheezing, pulmonary edema, CHF, and death
Betaxolol (Betoptic)		• Useful in treating glaucoma in patients with a history of CHF, asthma, or other conditions where β_2 blockade is contraindicated	• Limited side effects because it is cardioselective

*Eye drops must be used with care because they can cause lethal complications, such as hypertensive crisis and ventricular arrhythmias.

CLINICALLY IMPORTANT STRUCTURES OF THE EYE AND THEIR RECEPTORS

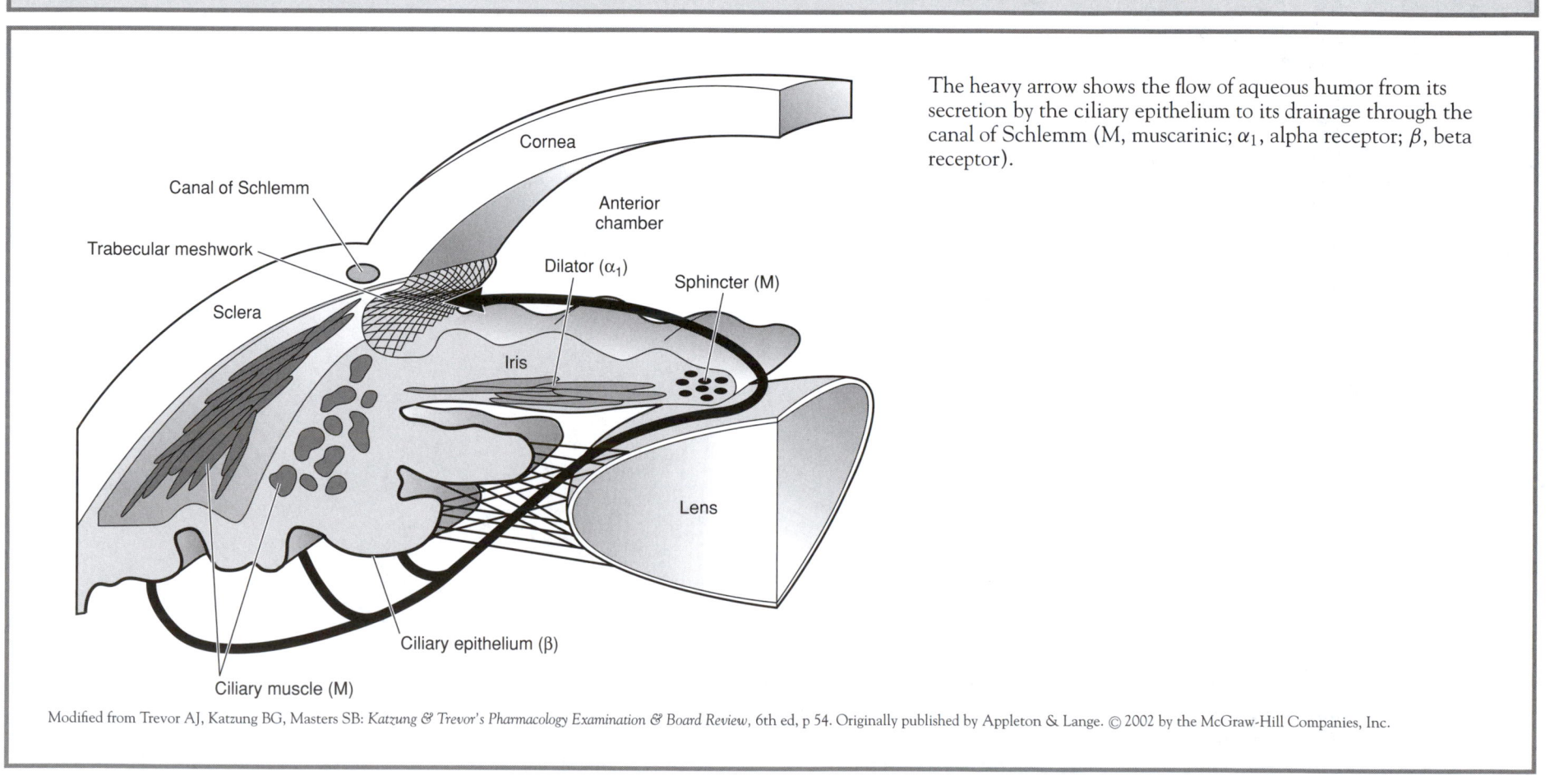

The heavy arrow shows the flow of aqueous humor from its secretion by the ciliary epithelium to its drainage through the canal of Schlemm (M, muscarinic; α_1, alpha receptor; β, beta receptor).

CHAPTER 4
PSYCHIATRIC MEDICATIONS

TERMS TO LEARN

Akathisia	An inner sense of restlessness.
Central Serotonin Syndrome	Caused by overactivation of central 5-HT receptors; symptoms include abdominal pain, diarrhea, sweating, fever, tachycardia, hypertension, delirium, myoclonus; can induce cardiovascular shock and death.
Delirium Tremors (DTs)	Autonomic instability, hallucinations, tremor, hypertension, tachycardia, and risk of seizures associated with cessation of alcohol ingestion.
Dyskinesias	Abnormal involuntary movement.
Extrapyramidal Syndrome (EPS)	Parkinson-like syndrome, akathisias, and dystonias.
Neuroleptic Malignant Syndrome (NMS)	Characterized by muscular rigidity, fever, and autonomic instability; associated with the use of neuroleptic medications (eg, haloperidol).
Tardive Dyskinesia (TD)	Syndrome of involuntary choreoathetoid movements associated with chronic use of neuroleptic medications; typically involves mouth, face, limbs, and trunk.
Trigeminal Neuralgia	Sharp, stabbing pain that occurs in one or more divisions of the trigeminal nerve.
Wernicke-Korsakoff Syndrome	Neurologic disorder caused by thiamine deficiency; often seen in chronic alcoholic patients; symptoms include confusion, ataxia, and memory impairment.

I. Antipsychotics

CLASSIFICATION OF ANTIPSYCHOTICS

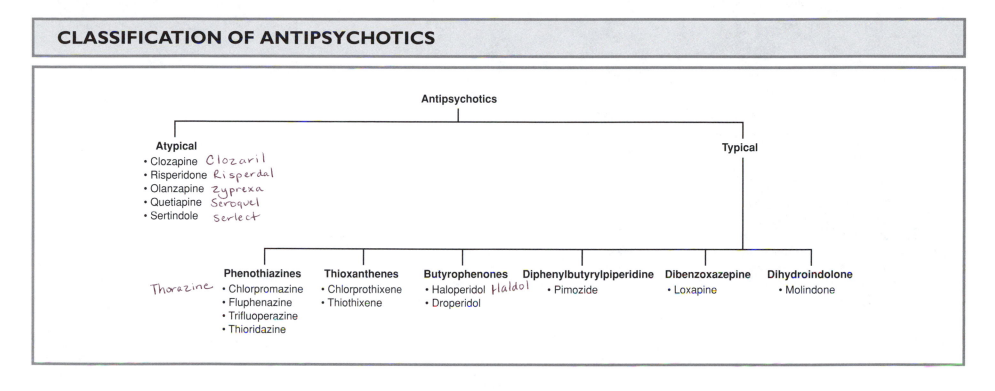

Antipsychotics

Atypical
- Clozapine   *Clozaril*
- Risperidone *Risperdal*
- Olanzapine *Zyprexa*
- Quetiapine *Seroquel*
- Sertindole *Serlect*

Typical

Phenothiazines   *Thorazine*
- Chlorpromazine
- Fluphenazine
- Trifluoperazine
- Thioridazine

Thioxanthenes
- Chlorprothixene
- Thiothixene

Butyrophenones
- Haloperidol *Haldol*
- Droperidol

Diphenylbutyrylpiperidine
- Pimozide

Dibenzoxazepine
- Loxapine

Dihydroindolone
- Molindone

TYPICAL ANTIPSYCHOTICS

Drug	Pharmacokinetics		Mechanism of Action	Clinical Uses	Drawbacks and Side Effects
Phenothiazines					
Chlorpromazine (Thorazine)	• **A:** IM, IV, and PO	• **D:** Widely distributed; crosses the BBB	• Blocks dopamine D$_2$ post synaptic receptor	• Treatment of schizophrenia	• Sedation
Fluphenazine (Prolixin, Permitil)	• **A:** IM, PO, and SC	• **M:** Hepatic metabolism (extensive first-pass metabolism)		• Treatment of psychotic features associated with other mental illnesses	• EPS
Trifluoperazine (Stelazine)	• **A:** IM and PO	• **E:** Parent drugs and metabolites excreted in urine and feces (thioxanthenes primarily excreted in urine)		• Treatment of positive symptoms (ie, hallucinations, delusions, thought broadcasting, etc)	• TD
Thioridazine (Mellaril)	• **A:** PO				• NMS
					• Strongest autonomic effects (peripheral α_1-blockade produces postural hypotension M$_2$-receptor blockade produces typical anticholinergic side effects, including urinary retention, constipation, dry mouth, blurry vision, etc)
					• D$_2$-receptor blockade effects (eg, hyperprolactinemia, gynecomastia, amenorrhea, galactorrhea, infertility)
					• Photosensitivity
					• Corneal deposits photosensitivity
					• Corneal deposits
Thioxanthenes					
Chlorprothixene (Taractan)	• **A:** IM and PO				• TD
					• NMS
Thiothixene (Navane)	• **A:** PO				• D$_2$-receptor blockade effects
					• Cardiotoxicity

Butyrophenones

| Haloperidol (Haldol) | • **A:** IM, IV, and PO | • EPS
• NMS
• TD
• D_2-receptor blockade effects |
| Droperidol (Inapsine) | • **A:** IM and IV | |

Diphenylbutyrylpiperidine

| Pimozide (Orap) | • **A:** PO | • TD
• NMS
• D_2-receptor blockade effects |

Dibenzoxazepine

| Loxapine (Loxitane) | • **A:** IM and PO | • TD
• NMS
• D_2-receptor blockade effects |

Dihydroindolone

| Molindone (Moban) | • **A:** PO | • TD
• NMS
• D_2-receptor blockade effects |

ATYPICAL ANTIPSYCHOTICS

Drug	Pharmacokinetics	Mechanism of Action	Clinical Uses and General Information	Drawbacks and Side Effects
Clozapine (Clozaril)	• **A:** PO; readily absorbed • **B:** Highly protein bound • **D:** Widely distributed; crosses the BBB • **M:** Hepatic metabolism (extensive first-pass metabolism) • **E:** Metabolites excreted in the urine ☞ ACROS Q	• Antagonism of D_4, α_1, 5-HT_2, and M receptors • Minimal antagonism H_1 receptors • Greater antagonism at 5-HT_2 than D_2 receptors • Minimally antagonistic on D_2 receptors	• Treatment of schizophrenia • Treatment of psychotic features associated with other mental illnesses • Given only to patients who are refractory to other antipsychotic drugs • Minimal EPS • Treatment of the negative symptoms of schizophrenia (ie, mutism, thought blocking, avolition, flattened affect, etc) • Produce less neurologic side effects than typical antipsychotics because of low potency at D_2 receptors • Less tendency to produce TD	• Agranulocytosis • Seizures • Anticholinergic side effects • Paradoxically produces drooling and excessive salivation • Sedation
Risperidone (Risperdal)	**A**typical antipsychotics **C**ross BBB **R**educed potency at D_2 **O**ral Administration **S**chizophrenia Tx **Q**uivering side effects reduced	• Antagonism of D_2 and 5-HT_2 receptors • Minimal antagonism of α_1, H_1, and M receptors • No effect on D_4 receptors	• Treatment of schizophrenia • Treatment of psychotic features associated with other mental illness • Risperidone has minimal EPS with low doses • Olanzapine and quetiapine have minimal EPS	• EPS with high doses • Hypotension with high doses
Olanzapine (Zyprexa)	**A**typical antipsychotics **C**lozapine **R**isperidone **O**lanzapine **S**ertinodole **Q**uetiapine	• Antagonism of 5-HT_2 receptors • Minimal antagonism of D_2, α_1, H_1, and M receptors • No effect on D_4 receptors	• Olanzapine and quetiapine are effective against both negative and positive symptoms associated with schizophrenia • Treatment of the negative symptoms of schizophrenia (ie, mutism, thought blocking, avolition, flattened affect, etc)	• Anticholinergic side effects • Weight gain

| Quetiapine (Seroquel) | • Antagonism of 5-HT$_2$ receptors
• Minimal antagonism of D$_2$, α_1, H$_1$, and M receptors
• No effect on D$_4$ receptors | • Produce less neurologic side effects than typical antipsychotics because of low potency at D$_2$ receptors
• Less tendency to produce TD | • Weight gain (less than with olanzapine) |
| Sertindole (Serlect) | • Antagonism 5-HT$_2$ > D$_2$ receptors
• Minimal antagonism of α_1 receptors
• No effect on D$_4$, H$_1$, and M receptors | | • Prolongation of the QT interval |

ATYPICAL ANTIPSYCHOTICS: MECHANISMS OF ACTION AT RECEPTOR SITES

Drug	Receptor					
	D$_2$	**D$_4$**	**5-HT$_2$**	**M**	**H$_1$**	**α_1**
Clozapine	Minimally antagonistic	Antagonistic	Antagonistic	Antagonistic	Minimally antagonistic	Antagonistic
Risperidone	Antagonistic	No effect	Antagonistic	Minimally antagonistic		Minimally antagonistic
Olanzapine	Minimally antagonistic	No effect	Antagonistic	Minimally antagonistic		
Quetiapine						
Sertindole	Antagonistic, but less so than on 5-HT$_2$	No effect	Antagonistic	No effect	No effect	

II. Antidepressants

CLASSIFICATION OF ANTIDEPRESSANTS

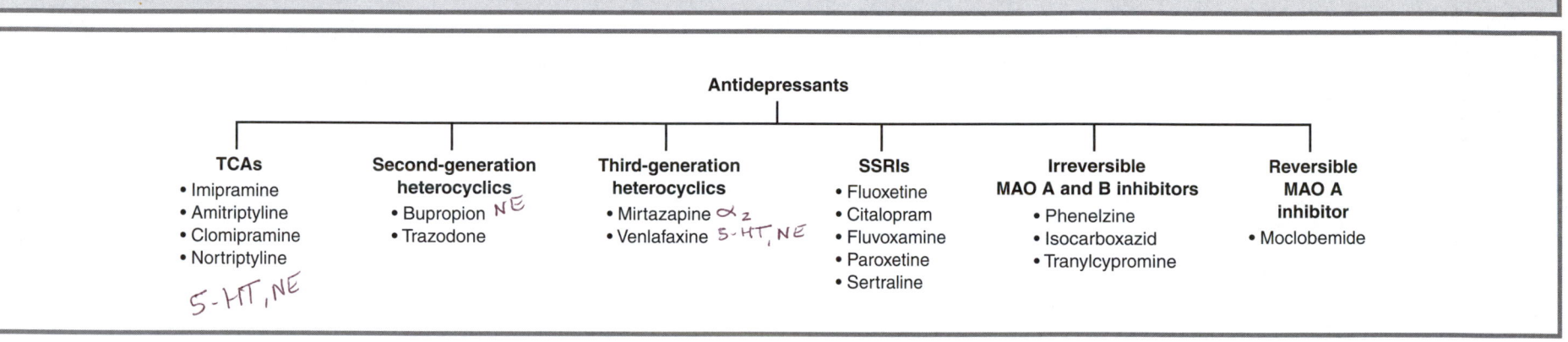

Antidepressants

TCAs
- Imipramine
- Amitriptyline
- Clomipramine
- Nortriptyline

5-HT, NE

Second-generation heterocyclics
- Bupropion NE
- Trazodone

Third-generation heterocyclics
- Mirtazapine α_2
- Venlafaxine 5-HT, NE

SSRIs
- Fluoxetine
- Citalopram
- Fluvoxamine
- Paroxetine
- Sertraline

Irreversible MAO A and B inhibitors
- Phenelzine
- Isocarboxazid
- Tranylcypromine

Reversible MAO A inhibitor
- Moclobemide

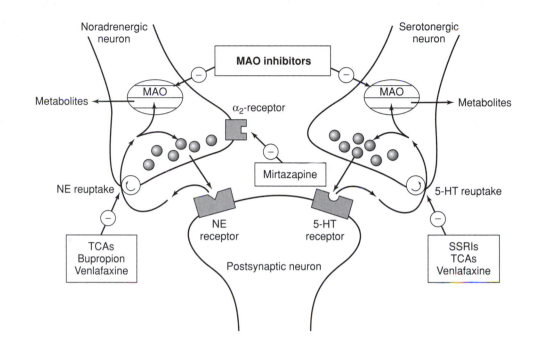

Many antidepressants may require administration for a number of weeks before achieving clinical efficacy.

Modified from Trevor AJ, Katzung BG, Masters SB: *Katzung & Trevor's Pharmacology Examination & Board Review*, 6th ed, p 270. Originally published by Appleton & Lange. © 2002 by the McGraw-Hill Companies, Inc.

TRICYCLIC ANTIDEPRESSANTS

Drug	Pharmacokinetics	Mechanism of Action	Clinical Uses	Drawbacks and Side Effects
Imipramine (Tofranil) Amitriptyline (Elavil) Clomipramine (Anafranil) Nortriptyline (Pamelor)	• **A:** PO; incompletely absorbed from the GI tract; imipramine and amitriptyline also available in IM form • **D:** High volume of distribution • **B:** Highly bound to plasma proteins • **M:** Significant hepatic first-pass metabolism; hydroxylated in the liver prior to excretion • **E:** Metabolites excreted in urine and feces	• Inhibit NE and 5-HT reuptake • Increase in synaptic NE and 5-HT	• Chronic pain disorders • Panic disorders • Enuresis (imipramine) • OCD (clomipramine)	• Contraindicated in patients with heart disease (due to conduction abnormalities); epilepsy (due to lower seizure threshold) and narrow-angle glaucoma • Cardiotoxicity including quinidine-like cardiac conduction block • Anticholinergic side effects • Sympathomimetic effects • Mania • Hypotension due to α_1 blockade • Sexual dysfunction • Sedation • Overdose associated with coma, cardiotoxicity, and convulsions (3Cs)

SECOND- AND THIRD-GENERATION HETEROCYCLICS

Drug	Pharmacokinetics	Mechanism of Action	Clinical Uses and General Information	Drawbacks and Side Effects
Second-Generation Heterocyclic				
Bupropion (Wellbutrin)	• **A:** PO; rapid absorption from GI tract • **M:** Extensive hepatic metabolism produces active metabolites • **E:** Metabolites excreted in urine and feces	• Inhibits NE reuptake • Weakly inhibits DA reuptake	• Depression • Adjunctive therapy in smoking cessation	• Dizziness • Dry mouth • Sweating • Tremor • Aggravation of psychosis • Potential seizure risk at high doses
Trazodone (Desyrel)	• **A:** PO; well absorbed from GI tract • **M:** Extensive hepatic metabolism • **E:** Majority of metabolites excreted in urine	• Inhibits 5-HT reuptake • Some 5-HT receptor antagonism	• Depression • Anxiolytic	• Sedation (may be exploited for treatment of insomnia) • Dizziness • Priapism
Third-Generation Heterocyclic				
Mirtazapine (Remeron)	• **A:** PO • **M:** Hepatic metabolism by P450 enzymes • **E:** Metabolites excreted in urine and feces	• α_2-Autoreceptor blocker • Inhibits autoregulation leading to increased NE and 5-HT release	• Depression • Anxiolytic	• Sedation (may be exploited for treatment of insomnia) • Weight gain • Dry mouth
Venlafaxine (Effexor)	• **A:** PO; well absorbed from GI tract • **M:** Extensive first-pass hepatic metabolism by P450 enzymes to active metabolite • **E:** Parent drug and metabolites excreted in urine	• Inhibit NE and 5-HT reuptake	• Depression • Less anticholinergic side effects than TCAs • No cardiotoxicity • No effect on seizure threshold	• Inhibitor of cytochrome P450 enzymes • Nausea • Headache • Insomnia • Sexual disturbances • Hypertension

SELECTIVE SEROTONIN REUPTAKE INHIBITORS

Drug	Pharmacokinetics	Mechanism of Action	Clinical Uses and General Information	Drawbacks and Side Effects
Fluoxetine (Prozac) Citalopram (Celexa) Fluvoxamine (Luvox) Paroxetine (Paxil) Sertraline (Zoloft)	• **A:** PO; well absorbed • **M:** Hepatic metabolism by P450 enzymes • **E:** Majority of metabolites excreted in urine; remainder in feces	• Inhibit 5-HT reuptake	• Depression • OCD (except citalopram) • Panic disorders • Less risk of cardiotoxicity than TCAs • Less toxic than TCAs in overdose	• Inhibitors of cytochrome P450 enzymes (numerous drug interactions); citalopram has least effect on enzymes • GI side effects (nausea, vomiting, diarrhea) • Sexual dysfunction • Central serotonin syndrome • Withdrawal syndrome (nausea, dizziness, anxiety, and tremors) • EPS may occur early in treatment • Seizures with overdose

MONOAMINE OXIDASE INHIBITORS

Drug	Pharmacokinetics	Mechanism of Action	Clinical Uses and General Information	Drawbacks and Side Effects
Noncompetitive, Irreversible Monoamine Oxidase (MAO) A and B Inhibitors				
Phenelzine (Nardil) Isocarboxazid (Marplan) Tranylcypromine (Parnate)	• **A:** PO; rapidly absorbed from GI tract • **M:** Hepatic metabolism • **E:** Metabolites excreted in urine	• Inhibits MAO A and B • Increases presynaptic stores of NE, DA, and 5-HT	• Atypical depression • Panic disorders • Limited usefulness because of side effect profile, including dietary restrictions	• Contraindicated with drugs rich in amines or that elevate synaptic amines including sympathomimetics like amphetamines, cold medicines, SSRIs, TCAs, and L-dopa; coadministration can cause a hypertensive crisis • Restrictive diet excluding foods rich in tyramine and other sympathomimetic amines • Sleep disturbances • Weight gain • Hypotension • Sexual disturbances (phenelzine) • Similar side effects to TCAs
Reversible Inhibitor of MAO A				
Moclobemide (Manerix)	• **A:** PO • **M:** Extensive hepatic metabolism • **E:** Metabolites excreted in urine	• Inhibit MAO A • Increases presynaptic stores of NE, DA, and 5-HT	• No dietary restrictions	• Insomnia • Dry mouth • Dizziness • Headache

III. Mood Stabilizing Agents

MOOD STABILIZING AGENTS: DRUG FACTS

Drug	Pharmacokinetics	Mechanism of Action	Clinical Uses	Drawbacks and Side Effects
Lithium (Lithobid, Eskalith)	• **A:** PO; completely absorbed from GI tract in about 8 hours; peak plasma concentration ~2–4 hours after an oral dose • **D:** In ECF with gradual accumulation; slow passage through BBB (CSF concentration 40% of plasma concentration) • **E:** ~95% eliminated in urine (one-third to two-third eliminated during initial 6–12 hours followed by a slow phase over 10–14 days)	• Not well defined • May decrease availability of IP$_3$ and DAG second messengers	• Acute mania • Prevention of recurrent bipolar affective illness	• Narrow therapeutic window (requires frequent monitoring) • Tremor • Sedation • Ataxia • Aphasia • Polydipsia/polyuria • Reversible nephrogenic diabetes insipidus • Edema • Acne • Leukocytosis • Benign thyroid enlargement • Use during pregnancy associated with congenital cardiac anomalies (ie, Ebstein's anomaly)

| Carbamazepine (Tegretol) | • **A:** PO; variable rate of absorption; peak blood levels 6–8 hours after administration
• **B:** 70% binding to plasma proteins
• **D:** Slow
• **M:** Hepatic metabolism by P450 enzymes (induces self-metabolism)
• **E:** Parent drug and metabolites excreted in urine | • Blocks Na$^+$ channels | • Anticonvulsant with antimanic properties (acute and prophylactic treatment of mania)
• Drug of choice for partial seizures
• Generalized tonic-clonic seizures
• Trigeminal neuralgia | • Contraindicated in pregnancy (neural tube defects)
• Diplopia
• Ataxia
• GI upset
• Induces microsomal enzymes (induces self-metabolism)
• CNS and respiratory depression with overdose
• Erythematous skin rash
• Aplastic anemia and agranulocytosis |
| Sodium valproate (Depakene, Depacon) | • **A:** PO; absorbed well; peak blood levels ~1–6 hours (enteric coated preparation is absorbed in basic pH of small intestine, decreasing nausea and stomach cramps)
• **B:** 80% serum protein binding
• **D:** Ionized at physiologic pH so distribution is confined to the ECF
• **M:** Via P450 system and mitochondrial β oxidation systems; yields many active metabolites
• **E:** $t_{1/2}$ 10–12 hours; Majority excreted as metabolites in urine | • Not well defined | • Anticonvulsant with antimanic properties (acute and prophylactic treatment) | • Contraindicated in pregnancy (neural tube and cardiovascular defects)
• GI distress
• Tremor
• Weight gain
• Hair loss
• Benign thrombocytopenia
• Hepatotoxicity |

IV. Receptor-Specific Drugs

CLASSIFICATION OF GABAERGIC AGENTS

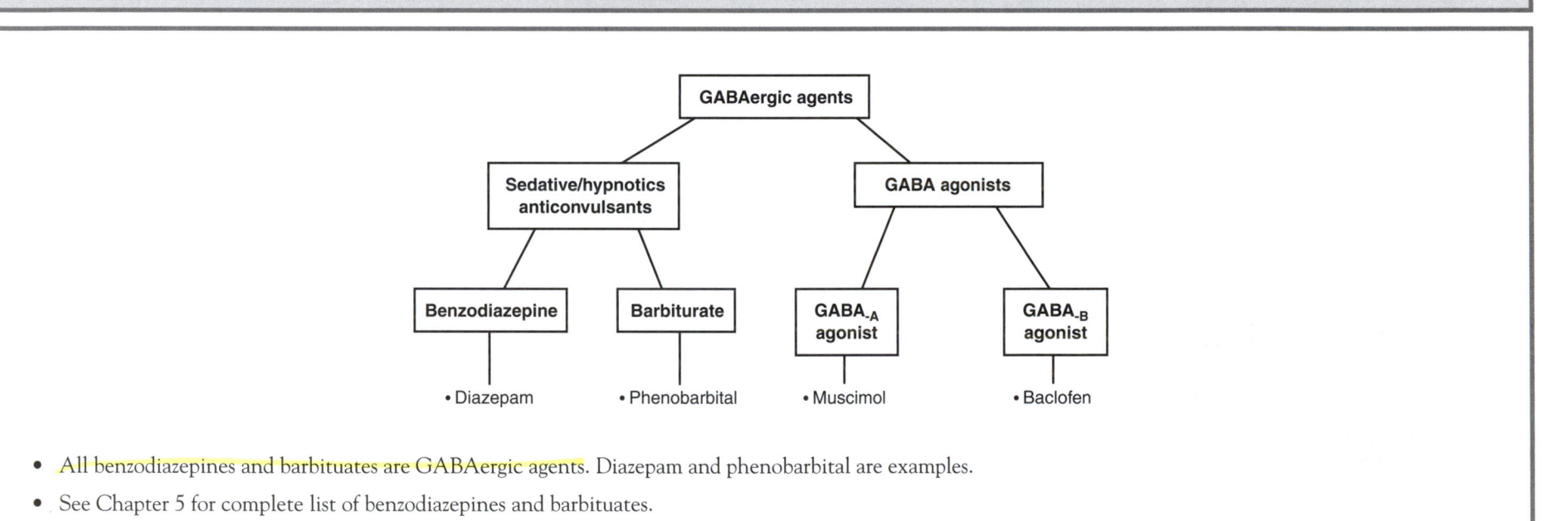

- All benzodiazepines and barbituates are GABAergic agents. Diazepam and phenobarbital are examples.
- See Chapter 5 for complete list of benzodiazepines and barbituates.

GABAERGIC AGENTS

Drug	Class	Pharmacokinetics	Mechanism of Action	Clinical Uses and General Information	Drawbacks and Side Effects
Diazepam (Valium)	• Benzodiazepine	• **A:** IM, IV, and PO; rapidly absorbed from GI tract • **B:** Highly bound to plasma proteins • **D:** Widely distributed; crosses BBB • **M:** Hepatic metabolism • **E:** Metabolites excreted in urine	• Increases the frequency of chloride channel openings by GABA at GABA-A receptor	• Anxiolytic • Anticonvulsant • Sedative/hypnotic • Skeletal muscle relaxant • Anesthesia	• Respiratory and cardiovascular depression (can be lethal in overdose) • Physiologic dependence • Tolerance
Phenobarbital (Solfoton)	• Barbiturate	• **A:** IM, IV, and PO; rapidly absorbed from GI tract • **D:** Widely distributed; crosses BBB • **M:** Hepatic metabolism; most metabolites are inactive • **E:** Metabolites excreted in urine	• Prolongs the duration of chloride channel openings by GABA at GABA-A receptor	• Anticonvulsant • Sedative/hypnotic	
Muscimol	• GABA-A agonist	• **A:** PO	• Opens chloride channel at GABA receptor	• Treatment of TD	• Clinical use limited by behavioral side effects
Baclofen (Lioresal)	• GABA-B agonist	• **A:** Intrathecal and PO; rapidly absorbed from GI tract • **M:** Slight degree of hepatic metabolism • **E:** Majority excreted unchanged in urine	• MOA is unknown; seems to inhibit afferent pathways in the spinal cord	• Skeletal muscle relaxant (through action in the CNS) • Less sedating than diazepam	• Drowsiness • Increases seizures in patients with epilepsy • Respiratory depression • Coma

DRUGS THAT ACT AT THE NMDA RECEPTOR

Drug	Pharmacokinetics	Mechanism of Action	Clinical Use	Drawbacks and Side Effects
Ketamine	• **A:** IV • **D:** Rapidly distributed; crosses BBB • **M:** Hepatic metabolism • **E:** In urine and feces	• Antagonist of glutamic acid • Blocks the NMDA receptor cation channel	• Dissociative anesthetic • Side effects limit clinical use	• Disorientation • Perceptual illusions • "Flashbacks" • Similar structure to PCP
Phencyclidine (PCP)	• Not applicable	• Blocks the NMDA receptor cation channel	• Psychomimetic drug of abuse	• Hallucinations • Nystagmus • Hypertension • Seizures

V. Treatment of Anxiety Disorders

THERAPEUTIC OPTIONS FOR VARIOUS ANXIETY DISORDERS

Disorder	Medication
Generalized anxiety	• Barbiturates (eg, phenobarbital; see Chapter 5) • Piperazines (eg, hydroxyzine; see Chapter 12) • Benzodiazepines (eg, diazepam; see Chapter 5) • Azapirones (eg, buspirone; see Chapter 5)
Symptomatic treatment of situational anxiety	• β-blockers (eg, propranolol; see Chapter 6)
Obsessive-compulsive disorder	• TCAs (eg, chlorimipramine) • SSRIs (eg, fluoxetine)
Phobic anxiety and panic attacks	• SSRIs • Tricyclic antidepressants (eg, imipramine) • Benzodiazepines (eg, diazepam; see Chapter 5) • Monoamine oxidase inhibitors • Benzodiazepines (eg, alprazolam; see Chapter 5)

VI. Drugs of Abuse

DRUGS OF ABUSE: THE FACTS

Drug	Mechanism of Action	Clinical Uses and Effects	Toxicity
Cannabinoid			
Marijuana	• Numerous active cannabinoids including THC • G-protein coupled receptor that acts via cAMP • Highest concentration of binding sites located in the basal ganglia, substantia nigra, pars reticulata, globus pallidus, hippocampus, and brainstem	• Dronabinol (controlled substance form of THC) used as an antiemetic and enhances appetite in HIV and cancer patients • Euphoria • "High" • Uncontrollable laughter • Alteration of time sense	• Tachycardia and hypotension associated with use • Reddened conjunctiva seen with chronic use
Hallucinogens			
Lysergic acid diethylamide (LSD)	• Specific MOA unknown • Appears to chemically resemble NE, DA, and 5-HT • Appears to alter 5-HT turnover	• Hallucinations • Altered mood • Poor judgement • Overactivity of sympathetic nervous system • Nausea • Weakness • Paresthesias • Not lethal	• Panic reactions • Flashbacks

Phencyclidine (PCP)	• Noncompetitive antagonist at the NMDA glutamate receptors	• Hallucinations • Disorientation • Detachment • Intoxication state resembles schizophrenia	• Acute psychosis • Overdose associated with hypertension and seizures; may be fatal
Inhalants			
Solvents, nitrous oxide, and nitrates	• Multiple MOAs • Not all well understood	• Psychoactive effects • Euphoria • Disinhibition	• Physiologic dependence • Hearing loss • Peripheral neuropathies • Brain damage • Bone marrow damage • Heart damage • Death
Opiate			
Heroin	• Acts at μ and δ opiate receptors in CNS	• Euphoria • Sedation • Analgesia	• Physiologic withdrawal syndrome (dilated pupils, watery eyes, anxiety, fever, diarrhea, weakness, depression) • Coma with respiratory depression and hypotension • Nalaxone can reverse overdose

Continued

DRUGS OF ABUSE: THE FACTS (Continued)

Drug	Mechanism of Action	Clinical Uses and Effects	Toxicity
Sedative			
Alcohol	• Specific MOA unknown • Appears to facilitate the action of GABA at the GABA$_A$ receptors • Inhibits the ability of glutamate to activate the NMDA receptor	• Sedation • Loss of inhibition • Impaired judgement • Slurred speech • Ataxia	• Additive CNS depression when coadministered with sedative-hypnotics, phenothiazines, and TCAs • Liver cirrhosis • GI (irritation and malnutrition) • CV (cardiomyopathy, increased incidence of MI) • Increased risk neoplasms • Fetal alcohol syndrome if ingested during pregnancy • Peripheral neuropathies • Wernicke-Korsakoff syndrome • DTs with cessation of use • Disulfiram (an aldehyde dehydrogenase inhibitor) induces noxious reactions in patients who coingest alcohol; utilized with behavioral therapy in an alcohol cessation program • Tolerance develops
Stimulants			
Caffeine	• Appears to work by blockade of presynaptic adenosine receptors	• Stimulation	• Withdrawal associated with lethargy, irritability, and headaches

Cocaine	• Blocks reuptake of DA, NE, and 5-HT • Strong action in DA pathways (pleasure pathways) of the CNS	• Vasoconstrictor and local anesthetic utilized clinically in ENT applications • Stimulation • Euphoria	• Strong physiologic dependence • Arrhythmias • Seizures • Respiratory depression • Hypertensive crisis (increases risk of CVA and MI) • Psychotic state with LTU
Methamphetamine (Speed)	• Increase the release of catecholamines (NE, DA, and 5-HT) • Weak inhibitor of block MAO • Possibly acts as a direct catecholamine agonist	• Mental alertness • Euphoria	• Strong physiologic dependence • Psychotic state associated with chronic use
Methylene Dioxymethamphetamine (MDMA, Ecstasy)	• Derivative of amphetamine	• Sensory enhancer • Disinhibition • Stimulation	• Damages 5-HT neurons with chronic use • Overdose resembles that of amphetamines
Nicotine	• Activates presynaptic and postsynaptic cholinergic nicotinic receptors • Triggers release of NE, EPI, and DA	• Mental alertness • Stimulation	• CNS stimulation (insomnia, tremors) associated with overdose • Physiologic dependence • Nicotine patches useful in managing withdrawal

CHAPTER 5
DRUGS AFFECTING NEUROLOGIC FUNCTION

I. DRUGS AFFECTING MOVEMENT

Classification of Drugs Used to Treat Movement Disorders

Protocol for Managing Parkinson's Disease

First-line Drugs for Parkinson's Disease

Second-line Drugs for Parkinson's Disease

Third-line Drugs for Parkinson's Disease

Treatment of Movement Disorders Other than Parkinson's Disease

II. DRUGS FOR ALZHEIMER'S DISEASE

Classification of Drugs Used for Alzheimer's Disease

Treating Alzheimer's Disease: Drug Facts

III. SEDATIVES AND HYPNOTICS

Sedatives and Hypnotics: Benzodiazepines

Sedatives and Hypnotics: Barbiturates

Other Sedatives and Hypnotics

IV. ANTIEPILEPTIC DRUGS

Mechanisms of Action of Antiepileptics

Antiseizure Drug Facts

Seizure Treatment Protocols

V. OPIOIDS

Opioids: Summary Table

Mechanism of Action of Opioids

Opioids: Strong Opioid Agonists

Opioids: Moderate to weak agonists, mixed agonist/antagonists, and antagonists

VI. DRUGS FOR THE TREATMENT OF MIGRAINES

Abortive and Prophylactic Therapy of Migraines

Abortive Antimigraine Therapy

Prophylactic Antimigraine Therapy

VII. ANTISPASTIC DRUGS

Mechanism of Action of Antispastic Drugs

Antispastic Drug Facts

VIII. LOCAL ANESTHETICS AND ADJUNCTIVE DRUGS

Local Anesthetics and Adjunctive Drugs: Summary Table

Classification of Local Anesthetics and Adjunctive Drugs

Local Anesthetics and Adjunctive Agents: Esters

Local Anesthetics and Adjunctive Agents: Amides and Other Nonesters

IX. GENERAL ANESTHETIC DRUGS

Classification of General Anesthetic Drugs

General Anesthetic Drugs: Inhaled

General Anesthetic Drugs: Intravenous Nonopioids

General Anesthetic Drugs: Intravenous Opioids

Four components, four stages, and four keys to anesthesia

Nonanesthetic drugs used during general anesthesia

X. NEUROMUSCULAR BLOCKERS

Neuromuscular Blockers: Summary Table

Nondepolarizing and Depolarizing Neuromuscular Blockers

Blepharospasm	Eyelid spasm.
Blood-to-Gas Partition Coefficient (B/G Coefficient)	An expression of solubility or the tendency of dissolved gas to come out of solution (ie, blood); low values indicate a fast-acting anesthetic.
Dysphagia	Difficulty swallowing.
Ergotism	Vasoconstriction leading to limb ischemia, gangrene, hypertension, and CNS disturbances; associated with the ingestion of ergots.
Lennox-Gastaut Syndrome	Childhood epileptic encephalopathy; syndrome of severe seizures, mental retardation, and characteristic EEG pattern.
Minimum Alveolar Concentration (MAC)	An expression of the concentration of inhaled anesthetic needed to keep 50% of patients from moving in response to surgical stimulus. Because it is a statistical measurement, all anesthetics are titrated until they produce the desired effect.
Pneumothorax	Air in the intrapleural space.
Strabismus	Nonparallel visual axis of the eyes.
West's Syndrome	Infantile spasms; age-specific form of generalized epilepsy.

I. Drugs Affecting Movement

CLASSIFICATION OF DRUGS USED TO TREAT MOVEMENT DISORDERS

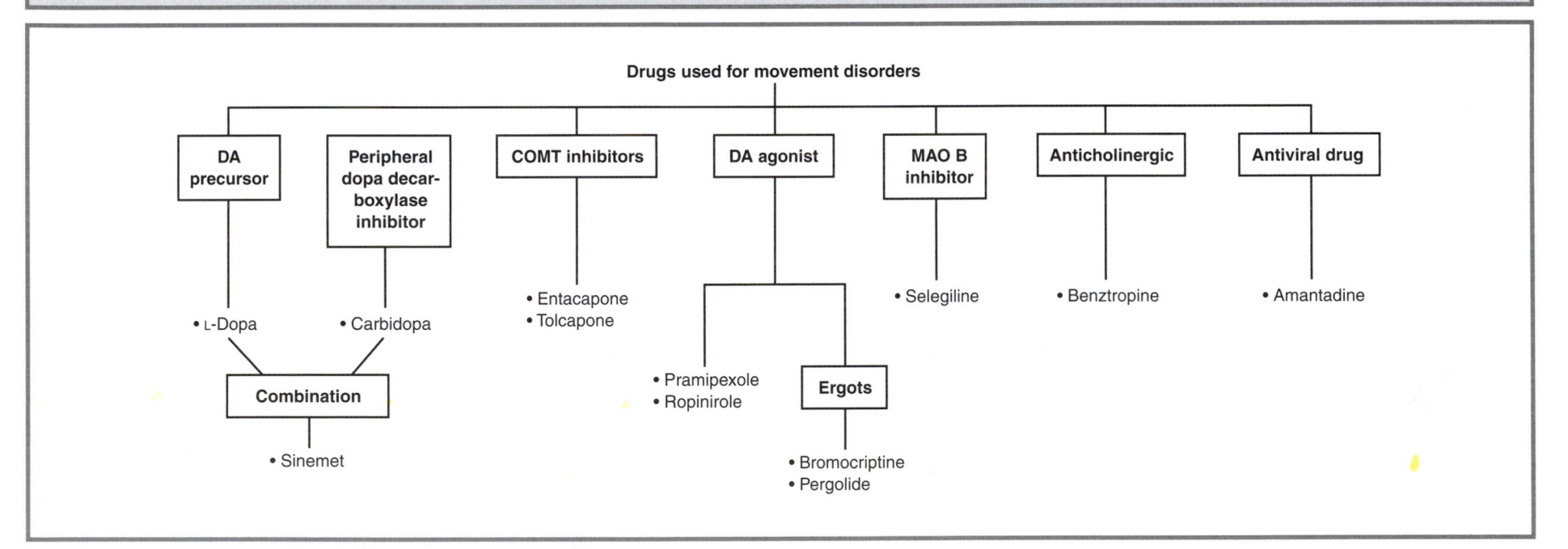

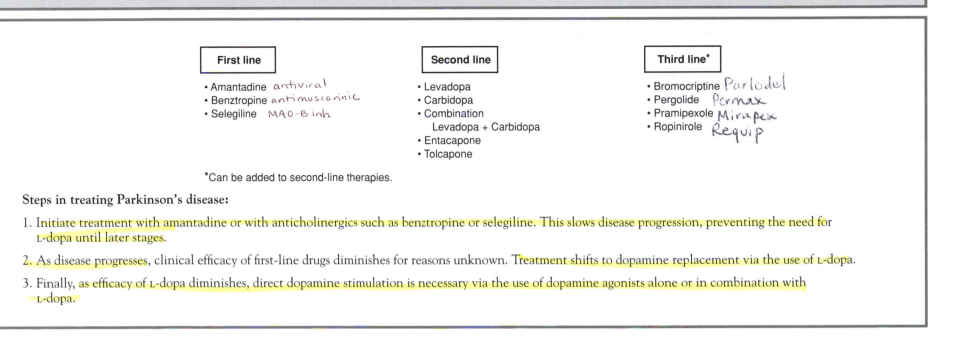

First line

- Amantadine *antiviral*
- Benztropine *antimuscarinic*
- Selegiline *MAO-B inh*

Second line

- Levadopa
- Carbidopa
- Combination
  Levadopa + Carbidopa
- Entacapone
- Tolcapone

Third line*

- Bromocriptine *Parlodel*
- Pergolide *Permax*
- Pramipexole *Mirapex*
- Ropinirole *Requip*

*Can be added to second-line therapies.

Steps in treating Parkinson's disease:

1. Initiate treatment with amantadine or with anticholinergics such as benztropine or selegiline. This slows disease progression, preventing the need for L-dopa until later stages.

2. As disease progresses, clinical efficacy of first-line drugs diminishes for reasons unknown. Treatment shifts to dopamine replacement via the use of L-dopa.

3. Finally, as efficacy of L-dopa diminishes, direct dopamine stimulation is necessary via the use of dopamine agonists alone or in combination with L-dopa.

FIRST-LINE DRUGS FOR PARKINSON'S DISEASE

Drug	Pharmacokinetics	Mechanism of Action	Clinical Uses	Contraindications	Drawbacks and Side Effects
Amantadine (Symmetrel)	• **A:** PO • **E:** Unchanged in urine	• Antiviral drug used to treat influenza (inhibits viral uncoating) • Causes DA release in the striatum	• Initial therapy for Parkinson's disease • Transient benefits	• Patients with CHF • Patients who are prone to seizure	• CNS disturbances (restlessness, depression, irritability, hallucinations, confusion) • GI disturbances (nausea, constipation, dry mouth) • Toxic psychosis with overdose
Benztropine (Cogentin)	• **A:** PO, IM, and IV; well absorbed • Remaining pharmacokinetics not well understood	• Antimuscarinic	• Treatment of rigidity and tremors associated with Parkinson's disease • Can be used to treat the parkinsonian symptoms that develop with the use of antipsychotics	• Children younger than 3 years • Patients with BPH • Obstructive GI disease • Narrow-angle glaucoma	• Nausea/vomiting • Antimuscarinic side effects
Selegiline (Eldepryl)	• **A:** PO; readily absorbed • **D:** Crosses BBB • **M:** Metabolized to active metabolites • **E:** In urine	• MAO B inhibitor • Prolongs action of DA by preventing its breakdown	• Enhances effect of L-dopa • May reduce on-off effects • May allow L-dopa dose reduction • May retard progression of Parkinson's disease	• Concomitant use with meperidine, TCAs, and SSRIs	• May increase adverse effects of L-dopa • Only selective MAO B inhibitor should be used with L-dopa because nonselective MAO inhibitors with L-dopa can cause a hypertensive crisis • Also blocks MAO A at high doses

SECOND-LINE DRUGS FOR PARKINSON'S DISEASE

Drug	Pharmacokinetics	Mechanism of Action	Clinical Uses	Contraindications	Side Effects
Levodopa (Larodopa)	• **A:** PO; rapidly absorbed from the small intestine • **D:** Crosses the BBB and is then converted to DA; only 1–3% of oral dose reaches the CNS • **M:** Metabolized in lumen of intestine, liver, kidney, and stomach • **E:** Majority excreted as metabolites in urine	• DA precursor • Increases concentration of available DA	• Treatment of DA-deficient state found in Parkinson's disease	• Pyridoxine (B$_6$) (a cofactor of DA β-hydroxylase) can exacerbate some side effects • Nonselective MAO inhibitors can cause hypertensive crisis • Coadministration with phenothiazines, which block DA receptors • Psychotic patients (exacerbates symptoms) • Patients with open-angle glaucoma or cardiac disease	• On-off phenomenon (fluctuations in clinical effects) **Early:** • Anorexia, nausea, and vomiting due to activation of chemoreceptor zones in the brain (decreased if doses are divided or if taken with meals—tolerance develops to this side effect) • Orthostatic hypotension • Arrhythmias (increased DA is converted to NE) • These side effects are less prominent when the drug is coadministered with a decarboxylase inhibitor **Late:** • Dyskinesia: facial grimacing, restless feet syndrome (increased incidence when combined with decarboxylase inhibitor; managed with drug holidays, dose reduction, or pallidotomy) • Psychiatric and behavioral side effects • Nightmares or anxiety

Continued

SECOND-LINE DRUGS FOR PARKINSON'S DISEASE (Continued)

Drug	Pharmacokinetics	Mechanism of Action	Clinical Uses	Contraindications	Side Effects
Carbidopa (Lodosyn)	• **A:** PO • **D:** Does not cross BBB	• Peripheral dopa decarboxylase inhibitor	• Used with L-dopa to prevent peripheral metabolism of L-dopa and increase the level in the CNS • Increases amount of dopa that reaches CNS	• Same as above	• Administered with L-dopa so side effect profile is same as above
Levodopa and Carbidopa (Sinemet)	• Same as above	• Combination of L-dopa and carbidopa	• Almost eliminates symptoms of nausea and vomiting • Cardiac side effect completely eliminated • Maintains more constant brain levels of L-dopa	• Narrow-angle glaucoma	• See above
Entacapone (Comtan)	• **A:** PO; rapidly absorbed • **D:** Does not cross BBB • **M:** Hepatic metabolism • **E:** Majority of metabolites excreted in feces	• COMT inhibitors • Prolong action of DA by preventing its breakdown	• Reduce clinical fluctuations in patients receiving L-dopa therapy	• Hypersensitivity	• Dyskinesias • Nausea • Confusion • Abdominal pain • Orthostatic hypotension • Sleep disturbances • Tolcapone is associated with hepatotoxicity
Tolcapone (Tasmar)	• **A:** PO; rapidly absorbed • **D:** Crosses BBB • **M:** Hepatic metabolism • **E:** Metabolites excreted in urine and feces			• Liver disease	

THIRD-LINE DRUGS FOR PARKINSON'S DISEASE

Drug	Pharmacokinetics	Mechanism of Action	Clinical Uses and General Information	Contraindications	Side Effects
Bromocriptine (Parlodel)	• **A:** PO; variable absorption • **M:** Hepatic metabolism • **E:** Majority of metabolites excreted in feces; remainder in urine	• Ergot • DA agonist • Preferential activity at the D_2 receptors	• Used to supplement levodopa and carbidopa as the combination loses efficacy • Treatment of hyperprolactinemia	• History of psychosis • Recent MI	• GI disturbances (nausea, vomiting, constipation, dyspepsia) • CV disturbances (postural hypotension, arrhythmias)
Pergolide (Permax)	• **A:** PO • **E:** Metabolites excreted in urine	• Ergot • DA agonist • Preferential activity at D_1 and D_2 receptors	• Used to supplement levodopa and carbidopa as combination loses efficacy • 10 times more potent than bromocriptine • Treatment of hyperprolactinemia		• Dyskinesias • Mental disturbances (confusion, hallucinations, delusions)
Pramipexole (Mirapex)	• **A:** PO; rapidly absorbed • **E:** Unchanged in urine	• DA agonist • Preferential activity at the D_3 receptors	• Monotherapy for mild Parkinson's disease • Combination therapy in advanced Parkinson's disease allows for decrease in L-dopa dose and decreases clinical fluctuations	• Hypersensitivity	• Postural hypotension • Fatigue • Sleep disturbances • Peripheral edema • Nausea • Constipation • Dyskinesias • Confusion
Ropinirole (Requip)	• **A:** PO • **M:** Hepatic metabolism by P450 enzymes • **E:** Majority excreted as metabolites in urine	• DA agonist • Preferential activity at the D_2 receptors			

TREATMENT OF MOVEMENT DISORDERS OTHER THAN PARKINSON'S DISEASE

Condition	Protocol
Physiologic postural tremor	• β_2-Blockers
Essential tremor	• β_1-Blockers • Primidone—prodrug, analogue of phenobarbital • Alprazolam—a benzodiazepine
Tourette's syndrome	• Haloperidol
Huntington's disease	• Phenothiazine • Butyrophenone • Reserpine

II. Drugs for Alzheimer's Disease

Acetylcholinesterase inhibitors are used to treat only the early stages of Alzheimer's disease. As the clinical efficacy of acetylcholinesterase inhibitors decreases, treatment shifts to a symptomatic approach, including standard psychiatric drugs such as antidepressants and antipsychotics (haloperidol, risperidone, and benzodiazepines).

CLASSIFICATION OF DRUGS USED FOR ALZHEIMER'S DISEASE

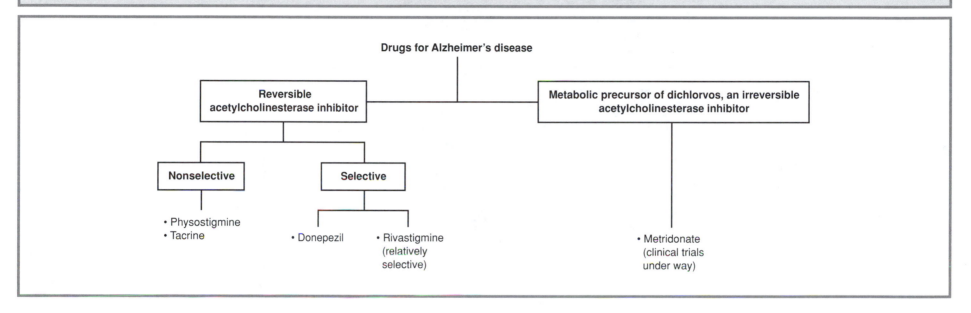

TREATING ALZHEIMER'S DISEASE: DRUG FACTS

Drug	Class/Mechanism of Action	Pharmacokinetics	Clinical Uses/Advantages	Side Effects
Physostigmine (Antilirium)	• Reversible, nonselective acetylcholinesterase inhibitor	• **A:** PO, IM, IV, and ophthalmic; well absorbed from all sites of administration • **D:** Enters CNS • $t_{1/2}$: 30 minutes–2 hours • **M:** Hydrolyzed by cholinesterases	• Used for Alzheimer's disease; discontinued because side effects outweighed benefits • Treatment of glaucoma	• Extensive cholinomimetic side effects
Tacrine (Cognex)	• Reversible, nonselective acetylcholinesterase and butyrylcholinesterase inhibitor	• **A:** PO; orally active • **D:** Enters CNS • $t_{1/2}$: Approximately 2 hours • **M:** Hepatic metabolism by P450 enzymes	• Enhances short-term memory and selective attention and language abilities in patients with Alzheimer's disease	• Nausea • Vomiting • Diarrhea • Abdominal cramps • Polyuria • Hepatotoxicity (limits clinical usefulness)
Donepezil (Aricept)	• Reversible, selective acetylcholinesterase inhibitor	• **A:** PO • **D:** Crosses BBB • $t_{1/2}$: 70 hours • **M:** Hepatic metabolism by P450 enzymes • **E:** Majority of metabolites excreted in urine; remainder in feces	• Treatment of mild to moderate Alzheimer's disease • Selective inhibition decreases side effects	• Nausea • Vomiting • Diarrhea • Loss of appetite • Muscle cramps • Fatigue

Rivastigmine (Exelon)	• Relatively selective and reversible acetylcholinesterase inhibitor	• **A:** PO • $t_{1/2}$: 10 hours • **M:** Extensive hydrolysis • **E:** Metabolites excreted in urine	• Improves global, behavioral, and cognition functioning	• Nausea • Vomiting • Anorexia • Dyspepsia • Asthenia
Metridonate	• Metabolic precursor of dichlorvos, an irreversible acetylcholinesterase inhibitor	• Not well defined	• Clinical trials underway	• Not well described

III. Sedatives and Hypnotics

As dosages increase, clinical results move from sedation to hypnosis to coma to death. Lower doses produce sedation, increases in dosages produce hypnosis, further increases produce coma, and additional increases produce death. Thus an abbreviated way to diagram dosages for sedatives and hypnotics is Sedation < Hypnosis < Coma < Death. ☞ SHoCkeD, where S stands for sedation, H for hypnotics and hypnosis, C for coma, and D for death.

SEDATIVES AND HYPNOTICS: BENZODIAZEPINES

Drug	Pharmacokinetics	Mechanism of Action	Clinical Uses and General Information	Side Effects
Diazepam (Valium)	• **A:** PO and IV; rapid oral absorption • **DOA:** Long • **M:** Hepatic metabolism to active metabolites • $t_{1/2}$: 20–80 hours • **E:** Renal excretion of metabolites	• Increase frequency of opening of Cl^- channel by GABA at $GABA_A$ receptor	• Anxiolytic • Treatment of insomnia • Sedation/amnesia before medical or surgical procedures • Treatment of epilepsy and seizure states • Control withdrawal from alcohol or other sedative/hypnotics • Muscular relaxation in specific neuromuscular disorders • Less tolerance and drug dependency than barbiturates	• Physiologic dependence • Formation of active metabolites (increases incidence of psychomotor dysfunction, including cognitive impairment, daytime sedation, and decreased psychomotor skills) • Amnesic effects • Additive CNS depression when combined with other sedative/hypnotics or alcohol
Flurazepam (Dalmane)	• **A:** PO • **DOA:** Long • **M:** Hepatic metabolism to active metabolites • $t_{1/2}$: 40–100 hours • **E:** Renal excretion of metabolites			

Quazepam (Doral)	• **A:** PO • **DOA:** Long • **M:** Hepatic metabolism to active metabolites • $t_{1/2}$: 30–100 hours • **E:** Renal excretion of metabolites	• Less reduction of REM • No induction of P450 system (less drug interactions) • Higher margin of safety and high therapeutic index • Less respiratory depression • Availability of flumazenil (a benzodiazepine competitive antagonist) in case of overdose
Alprazolam (Xanax)	• **A:** PO • **DOA:** Intermediate • **M:** Hepatic metabolism to active metabolites • $t_{1/2}$: 12–15 hours • **E:** Renal excretion of metabolites	
Estazolam (ProSom)	• **A:** PO • **DOA:** Intermediate • **M:** Hepatic metabolism to inactive metabolites • $t_{1/2}$: 10–24 hours • **E:** Renal excretion of metabolites	
Lorazepam (Ativan)	• **A:** PO and IV; slow oral absorption • **DOA:** Intermediate • **M:** Does not require hepatic metabolism • $t_{1/2}$: 10–20 hours • **E:** Renal excretion of metabolites	

Continued

SEDATIVES AND HYPNOTICS: BENZODIAZEPINES (Continued)

Drug	Pharmacokinetics	Mechanism of Action	Clinical Uses and General Information	Side Effects
Oxazepam	• **A:** PO; slow oral absorption • **DOA:** Intermediate • **M:** Does not require hepatic metabolism • $t_{1/2}$: 10–20 hours • **E:** Renal excretion of metabolites			
Temazepam (Restoril)	• **A:** PO; slow oral absorption • **DOA:** Intermediate • **M:** Does not require hepatic metabolism • $t_{1/2}$: 10–12 hours • **E:** Renal excretion of metabolites			
Triazolam (Halcion)	• **A:** PO; rapid oral absorption • **DOA:** Short • **M:** Hepatic metabolism to short acting active metabolite • $t_{1/2}$: 2–4 hours • **E:** Renal excretion of metabolites			

SEDATIVES AND HYPNOTICS: BARBITURATES

- Good hypnotic drugs have a fast onset of action.

- Good sedative drugs have a slow onset of action.

- Sedatives and hypnotics have an antiepileptic effect when a methyl group is attached to a *N* within the ring (eg, phenobarbital).

Drug	Pharmacokinetics	Mechanism of Action	Clinical Uses	Side Effects
Phenobarbital	- **A:** PO, IM, and IV - **DOA:** 6–12 hours - **OOA:** 20 minutes - **M:** Metabolized by the hepatic P450 system	- Increase duration of Cl^- channel opening by GABA at the GABA$_A$ receptor thereby depressing the reticular activating system - Performs the same action without GABA at high doses	- Sedative/hypnotic - Preanesthetic agent - Anticonvulsant (generalized tonic-clonic seizures)	- Death - CNS depression (additive effects with alcohol and other CNS depressants) - Rash, dermatitis - Acute toxicity with overdose (respiratory, CV, and CNS depression, renal failure)
Pentobarbital (Nembutal)	- **A:** PO, IM, IV, and rectal - **DOA:** 4–6 hours - **OOA:** 3 minutes - **M:** Metabolized by the hepatic P450 system		- Sedative/hypnotic - Coma induction in patients with status epilepticus or increased intracranial pressure	- Chronic toxicity (abuse and addiction, tolerance and dependency can lead to status epilepticus during withdrawal) - P450 induction (LTU causes induction of these enzymes, which leads to tolerance and decreased efficacy of other drugs as well)
Secobarbital (Seconal)	- **A:** PO, IM, IV, and rectal - **DOA:** 2–4 hours - **OOA:** 2 minutes - **M:** Metabolized by the hepatic P450 system		- Sedative/hypnotic - Preanesthetic agent	- Decreased REM time (causes rebound REM with anxiety following drug removal)
Thiopental (Pentothal)	- **A:** IV and rectal - **DOA:** 15–30 minutes - **OOA:** Few seconds - **M:** Metabolized by the hepatic P450 system		- Anesthesia induction - Supplement to regional anesthesia - Rapid sequence intubation	- May precipitate acute intermittent porphyria in susceptible patients - Treat overdose with diuresis and by making urine basic ($NaHCO_3$) to keep the molecules charged and increase urinary excretion

OTHER SEDATIVES AND HYPNOTICS

Drug	Pharmacokinetics	Mechanism of Action	Clinical Uses	Side Effects
Buspirone (Buspar)	• **A:** PO; well absorbed • **B:** >90% plasma protein binding • **M:** Hepatic metabolism to active metabolites	• 5-HT$_{1A}$ agonist	• Anxiety disorders • Nonsedating • Limited abuse potential • Does not potentiate CNS depressive effects of ethanol	• Tachycardia/palpitations • Nervousness • GI distress • Paresthesias • Requires weeks of administration to establish an anxiolytic effect
Chloral hydrate	• **A:** PO (liquid) • **M:** Prodrug, metabolized to trichloroethanol (active metabolite) by alcohol dehydrogenase	• Related to alcohol • Exact mechanism of action unclear	• Sedative/hypnotic used in the geriatric population because it does not decrease respiration as much as barbiturates and benzodiazepines	• Displaces coumarins from plasma binding proteins increasing its anticoagulant properties • Questionable carcinogenicity
Paraldehyde	• **A:** PO, rectal, or IV • **M:** Trimer of acetaldehyde that is metabolized to acetate; 60% of acetate enters Krebs cycle for metabolism and the other 40% is exhaled	• CNS depressant • Likely acts on the reticular activating system	• Anticonvulsant • For alcoholic and agitated psychiatric patients to calm them and help them sleep	• Foul tasting and smelling (smells like garlic) • Skin rash • Cough with IV administration • Drowsiness • Nausea and vomiting • Dizziness
Zolpidem (Ambien)	• **A:** PO • **M:** Rapid hepatic metabolism	• Nonbenzodiazepine that selectively binds to the benzodiazepine binding site on the GABA receptor	• Treatment of insomnia • Actions similar to benzodiazepines without the tolerance or dependency problems • Safer than benzodiazepines • Overdose can be treated with flumazenil	• Suppresses REM sleep at higher doses • Respiratory depression when large doses are combined with other sedative/hypnotics or alcohol

IV. Antiepileptic Drugs

MECHANISMS OF ACTION OF ANTIEPILEPTICS

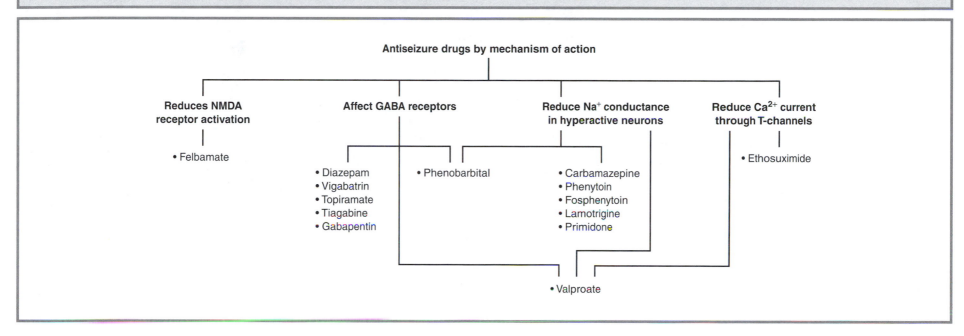

Antiseizure drugs by mechanism of action

Reduces NMDA receptor activation

- Felbamate

Affect GABA receptors

- Diazepam
- Vigabatrin
- Topiramate
- Tiagabine
- Gabapentin

- Phenobarbital

Reduce Na⁺ conductance in hyperactive neurons

- Carbamazepine
- Phenytoin
- Fosphenytoin
- Lamotrigine
- Primidone

Reduce Ca²⁺ current through T-channels

- Ethosuximide

- Valproate

ANTISEIZURE DRUG FACTS

Drug	Pharmacokinetics	Mechanism of Action	Clinical Uses	Side Effects
Diazepam (Valium)	• **A:** PO, IM, IV, and rectal • **M:** Hepatic metabolism to active metabolites • $t_{1/2}$: 20–80 hours • **E:** Metabolites excreted in urine	• Bind to benzodiazepine site on $GABA_A$ receptor and act to potentiate GABA's action by increasing frequency of opening of Cl^- channel • By enhancing GABAs action, they inhibit the onset or control the spread of seizures	• Status epilepticus • Also used as sedative/hypnotic	• Physiologic dependence • Formation of active metabolites (increases incidence of psychomotor dysfunction including cognitive impairment, daytime sedation, and decreased psychomotor skills) • Amnesic effects • Additive CNS depression when combined with other sedative/hypnotics or alcohol
Phenobarbital	• **A:** PO; absorbed completely • **D:** Enters the brain slowly • **B:** 50% binding to plasma proteins • $t_{1/2}$: Approximately 100 hours (in adults) • **M:** Liver; induces P450 system • **E:** Metabolites excreted in urine	• Enhances GABA's action at the $GABA_A$ receptor by increasing duration of Cl^- channel opening • Reduces Na^+ conductance • Blocks excitatory responses induced by glutamate	• Partial seizures • Generalized tonic-clonic seizures • Also used as a preanesthetic agent and sedative/hypnotic	• Sedation • Dependence • Tolerance • P450 induction • Additional information available in sedative hypnotic charts
Vigabatrin (Sabril)	• **A:** PO; rapidly absorbed • $t_{1/2}$: 6–8 hours • **E:** Majority excreted unchanged in urine	• Irreversible GABA-T inhibitor • Prolongs the action of GABA by inhibiting its degradation by GABA-T	• Partial seizures • West's syndrome • Clinical use is reserved for refractory patients due to side effect profile	• Agitation • Confusion • Drowsiness • Dizziness • Psychosis • Weight gain • LTU associated with irreversible visual field defects

Drug	Pharmacokinetics	Mechanism of Action	Indications	Side Effects
Topiramate (Topamax)	• **A:** PO; rapidly absorbed • **B:** 15% plasma protein binding • **E:** Unchanged in urine	• Potentiates GABA's effect • Blocks voltage gated Na^+ channels	• Partial seizures • Generalized seizures • Absence seizures • West's syndrome • Lennox-Gastaut syndrome	• Cognitive slowing • Confusion and nervousness • Dizziness • Fatigue and somnolence • Paresthesias • Renal stones • Weight loss
Tiagabine (Gabatril)	• **A:** PO • $t_{1/2}$: Very short (12 hours) • **M:** Hepatic metabolism • **E:** Majority of metabolites excreted in feces; remainder in urine	• Blocks neuronal and glial reuptake of GABA	• Adjunctive therapy of partial seizures	• Dizziness • Headaches • Drug interactions: may decrease valproate levels
Gabapentin (Neurontin)	• **A:** PO • **B:** Not significantly bound to plasma proteins • **E:** Unchanged in urine	• Enhances the release of GABA via an unknown mechanism	• Psychiatric disorders • Chronic pain • Epilepsy	• Behavioral changes in children • Leukopenia • Movement disorders • Sedation
Felbamate (Felbatol)	• **A:** PO • $t_{1/2}$: 20 hours • **E:** Majority excreted unchanged in urine	• Reduces NMDA receptor activation • Decreases excitation by competitively blocking strychnine insensitive glycine site on the NMDA receptor • Enhances GABA's action at the $GABA_A$ receptor	• Partial seizures • Useful for seizures associated with Lennox-Gastaut syndrome • Severe side effects limit clinical usefulness	• Hepatitis • Aplastic anemia • Drug interactions: felbamate increases phenytoin and valproate, decreases carbamazepine levels

Continued

ANTISEIZURE DRUG FACTS (Continued)

Drug	Pharmacokinetics	Mechanism of Action	Clinical Uses	Side Effects
Carbamazepine (Tegretol)	• **A:** PO • **B:** 75% binding to plasma proteins • **M:** Hepatic metabolism by P450 enzymes; induces P450 system (autoinduction) • **E:** Majority of metabolites excreted in urine; remainder in feces	• Reduce Na$^+$ conductance in hyperactive neurons	• Drug of choice for partial seizures • Generalized tonic-clonic seizures • Also used to treat trigeminal neuralgia and bipolar affective disorder	• Ataxia • Diplopia • Drowsiness • Drug interactions due to induction of hepatic enzymes • GI upset • Idiosyncratic blood dyscrasias • Teratogen • Vertigo
Phenytoin (Dilantin)	• **A:** PO, IM, and IV • **B:** Highly bound to serum proteins (>90%) • **M:** Metabolized by hepatic microsomal enzymes • **E:** In urine		• Partial seizures • Generalized tonic-clonic seizures • Status epilepticus	• Drug interactions: decreased by inducers of liver metabolism (eg, sulfonamides, valproate); increased by inhibitors of liver metabolism (ie, cimetidine, isoniazid) • Fosphenytoin is a prodrug of phenytoin with improved aqueous solubility • Nystagmus • Diplopia • Ataxia • Idiosyncratic rash • Gingival hyperplasia • Hirsutism • Vitamin D deficiency • Hypersensitivity reactions including Stevens-Johnson syndrome
Fosphenytoin (Cerebyx)	• **A:** IM and IV NO PO • **M:** Hepatic metabolism • **E:** Metabolites excreted in urine			

Lamotrigine (Lamictal)	• **A:** PO; complete absorption	• Monotherapy in partial seizure disorders	• Dizziness and ataxia
	• **B:** 55% binding to plasma proteins	• Absence and myoclonic seizures in children	• Sedation and somnolence
	• $t_{1/2}$: 24 hours	• Generalized tonic-clonic seizures	• Headache
	• **M:** Hepatic metabolism		• Diplopia
	• **E:** Majority of metabolites excreted in urine		• Nausea
			• Skin rash
			• Hepatotoxicity
			• Stevens-Johnson syndrome (1–2% of pediatric patients)
			• Drug interaction: valproate coadministration doubles lamotrigine's $t_{1/2}$ via inhibition of glucuronidation
Primidone (Mysoline)	• **A:** PO; completely absorbed from GI tract	• Partial seizures	• Similar toxicity profile to that of phenobarbital
	• **M:** Hepatic metabolism to two active antiepileptic agents (PEMA and phenobarbital)	• Generalized tonic-clonic seizures	
	• **E:** Metabolites excreted in urine		

Continued

ANTISEIZURE DRUG FACTS (Continued)

Drug	Pharmacokinetics	Mechanism of Action	Clinical Uses	Side Effects
Valproate (Depacon, Depakote)	• **A:** PO and IV; well absorbed • **B:** 90% binding to plasma proteins • **M:** Hepatic metabolism • **E:** Majority of metabolites excreted in urine	• Reduces Ca^{2+} current through T channels • Competitive GABA-T inhibitor • Reduces Na^+ conductance in hyperactive neurons	• Multiple actions give this its broad therapeutic action • Most seizure types	• May induce hepatotoxicity (worst in children older than 2 years) • Teratogen (may cause spina bifida) • Ataxia • GI distress • Sedation • Cognitive blunting (problem in school age kids)
Ethosuximide (Zarontin)	• **A:** PO; well absorbed • **B:** Very low protein binding • $t_{1/2}$: 40 hours • **M:** 50–75% metabolized by hepatic microsomal enzymes to inactive metabolites • **E:** Parent drug and metabolites excreted in urine	• Reduces Ca^{2+} current through T channels	• Absence (petit mal) seizures	• GI disturbances • Lethargy • CNS: headaches, dizziness • Rare occurrences of rashes • Drug interactions: coadministration with valproate increases ethosuxamide levels

SEIZURE TREATMENT PROTOCOLS

Seizure Type	Description	Protocol
Partial seizures	• Simple: seizure in a discrete region of the brain without altered consciousness • Complex: simple seizure with altered consciousness • Partial with secondary generalization: begins as a simple seizure and then spreads throughout the cortex	• Carbamazepine—drug of choice • Phenytoin • Valproate • Phenobarbital • Primidone • Adjuncts (used only if monotherapy is unsuccessful): lamotrigine, gabapentin, tiagabine, topirimate
Generalized seizures (grand mal) *tonic-clonic*	• Seizures that arise from bilateral brain hemispheres without focal onset • Accompanied by loss of consciousness	• Same drugs as those to treat partial seizures except valproate is the drug of choice
Petit mal seizures *absence*	• Brief lapses in consciousness without loss of postural control	• Ethosuximide • Valproate is drug of choice when tonic-clonic seizures are also present • Clonazepam is still used in some kids with petit mal or myoclonic seizures, not the drug of choice • Adjunct: lamotrigine
Myoclonic seizures	• Sudden, brief muscle contraction involving one part of the body	• Valproate • Some benzodiazepines
Infantile spasms (West's syndrome)	• Seizure disorder of early childhood or infancy • Usually occurs in the first year of life • Characterized by myoclonic seizures and mental retardation	• ACTH • Prednisone • Vigabatrine
Status epilepticus	• Prolonged seizure activity without recovery of consciousness or discrete seizures without regaining consciousness in the period between	Phenytoin or fosphenytoin with a benzodiazepine (diazepam or lorazepam)

V. Opioids

Endogenous opioids include dynorphins, enkephalins, and endorphins.

OPIOIDS: SUMMARY TABLE

General Pharmacokinetics	Mechanism of Action	Clinical Uses of Opioid Agonists	Adverse Effects			
			Acute Side Effects	Chronic Side Effects	Toxicities	Abstinence Syndrome
• Well absorbed via intramuscular, subcutaneous, and muscosal sites; PO administration often accompanied by extensive first-pass metabolism • Distribution depends on chemical properties of each opioid; some readily cross the BBB, all readily cross the placenta • Most undergo hepatic metabolism to polar metabolites • Renal excretion of polar metabolites	• MOA relies on endogenous receptors: • μ_1—analgesic receptors found supraspinally • μ_2—analgesic receptors found in the spinal cord, also mediate respiratory depression and GI transit depression • δ-unknown function in humans • κ_1—analgesic receptors found in the spinal cord • κ_3—analgesic receptors found supraspinally	• Analgesia: mild to moderate pain • Acute pulmonary edema: calms patient and slows respiration • MI: analgesic and sedative effects • Preanesthetic medication: sedative, analgesic • Anesthetic • Antitussive • Antidiarrheal	• Nausea and vomiting • Constipation • Mental clouding • Muscular rigidity • Euphoria • Dysphoria • Respiratory center depression • Miosis	• Tolerance • Cross tolerance throughout the class • Physiologic dependence	• Overdose leading to coma with respiratory depression and hypotension can be fatal • Additive CNS depression when combined with EtOH, sedative/hypnotics, anesthetics, antipsychotics, TCAs, or antihistamines	• Rhinorrhea and lacrimation • Yawning • Anxiety and hostility • Chills and gooseflesh • Muscle aches • Diarrhea

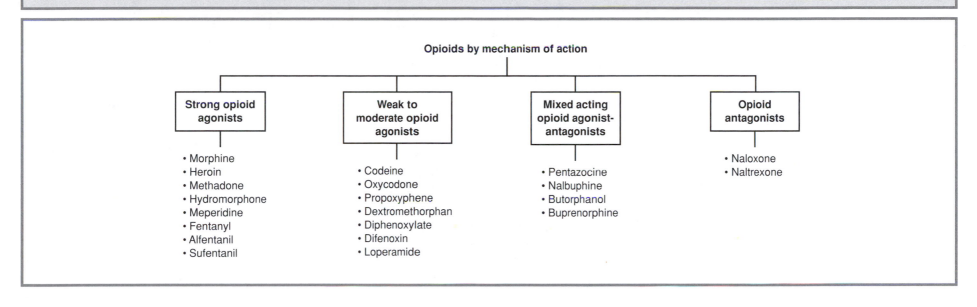

OPIOIDS: STRONG OPIOID AGONISTS

Drug	Receptor Effects			Pharmacokinetics	Clinical Uses	Side Effects
	μ	δ	κ			
Morphine (MS Contin, Duramorph)	• μ Agonist	• δ Agonist	• κ Agonist	• **A:** IV, IM, SC, PO, and rectal; poor oral availability • **M:** Produces three glucuronidated metabolites (only 6-OH is active), extensive first-pass metabolism after PO administration	• Analgesia • Sedation • Decreases perception of dyspnea in patients with pulmonary edema	• See summary table • Itching from histamine release
Heroin				• **A:** IV, PO, and intranasal • **M:** Prodrug of morphine with higher lipid solubility so crosses BBB easily	• Illicit drug of abuse	• See summary table • See Drugs of Abuse chart in Chapter 4 for additional information
Methadone (Dolophine)	• μ Agonist	• δ Agonist at high doses	• κ Agonist at high doses	• **A:** PO, IM, and SC • **DOA:** Longest acting opioid	• Heroin detoxification and maintenance therapy	• See summary table
Hydromorphone (Dilaudid)				• **A:** PO, IM, IV, SC, and rectal • **M:** Extensive first-pass metabolism after PO administration	• Analgesic	• See summary table • High abuse potential limits use

Meperidine (Demerol)	• **A:** PO, IM, IV, and SC • **M:** Metabolized to normeperidine; stimulates the hepatic microsomal system to up regulate its own metabolism	• Analgesic	• Contraindicated in epileptics • See summary table • Serotonin syndrome when combined with SSRIs or MAO inhibitors • Antimuscarinic side effects • Potential for causing seizures • Histamine release • Constipation less common
Fentanyl (Sublimaze, Duragesic)	• **A:** IM and IV (Sublimaze) and transdermal patch (Duragesic)	• Analgesic	• See summary table
Alfentanil (Alfenta)	• **A:** IV	• Analgesic • Less potent than fentanyl	
Sufentanil (Sufenta)	• **A:** IM, IV, and epidural	• Analgesic • 5–7 times the potency of fentanyl	

OPIOIDS: MODERATE TO WEAK AGONISTS, MIXED AGONIST/ANTAGONISTS, AND ANTAGONISTS

Drug	Receptor Effects			Pharmacokinetics	Clinical Uses	Side Effects
	μ	δ	κ			
Moderate to Weak Opioid Agonists						
Codeine	μ Agonist	δ Agonist at high doses	κ Agonist at high doses	• **A:** PO, IM, and SC • **D:** Readily crosses BBB • **M:** Prodrug converted to morphine	• Antitussive • Used as an analgesic when combined with aspirin or acetaminophen	• See summary table • Itching from histamine release
Oxycodone (Oxycontin)				• **A:** PO	• An analgesic when combined with aspirin (Percodan) or acetaminophen (Percocet)	• See summary table
Propoxyphene (Darvon)				• **A:** PO	• Limited clinical usefulness • An analgesic when combined with aspirin or acetaminophen	• See summary table • Deaths associated with abuse
Dextromethorphan (Sucrets, Robitussin DM)				• **A:** PO	• Antitussive	• See summary table less risk of side effects due to lower agonist qualities
Diphenoxylate (Lomotil)				• **A:** PO	• Treatment of diarrhea • Small amount of atropine added to prevent abuse	
Difenoxin (Motofen)				• **A:** PO		
Loperamide (Imodium)				• **A:** PO	• Treatment of diarrhea	

Mixed Agonist/Antagonists

Nalbuphine (Nubain)	μ Antagonist	No significant δ activity	κ Agonist	• **A:** IM, IV, and SC	• Analgesic • No abuse potential • Safer and used more often than pentazocine	• Sedation • Dizziness • Sweating • Nausea
Pentazocine (Talwin)	Partial μ agonist			• **A:** PO, IM, IV, and SC	• Analgesic	• Anxiety • Hallucinations
Butorphanol (Stadol)				• **A:** IM, IV, or nasal spray	• Analgesic • Low abuse potential	• Cause less respiratory depression than full agonist
Buprenorphine (Buprenex)			κ Antagonist	• **A:** IM and IV	• Analgesic • Heroin detoxification and maintenance therapy	• Physical dependence • Milder withdrawal symptoms

Opioid Antagonist

Naloxone (Narcan)	μ Antagonist	δ Antagonist	κ Antagonist	• **A:** IM, IV, and SC; poor oral efficacy • **DOA:** 1–2 hours	• Treatment of acute opioid overdose • Short-acting so repeated administration is required	• Can precipitate an intense abstinence syndrome in opioid-dependent patients
Naltrexone (Trexan)				• **A:** PO; well absorbed • **DOA:** 24–48 hours	• Treatment of acute opioid overdose • Adjunctive therapy in alcohol dependency programs	• LTU can cause hepatotoxicity • Can precipitate an intense abstinence syndrome in opioid-dependent patients

VI. Drugs for the Treatment of Migraines

ABORTIVE AND PROPHYLACTIC THERAPY OF MIGRAINES

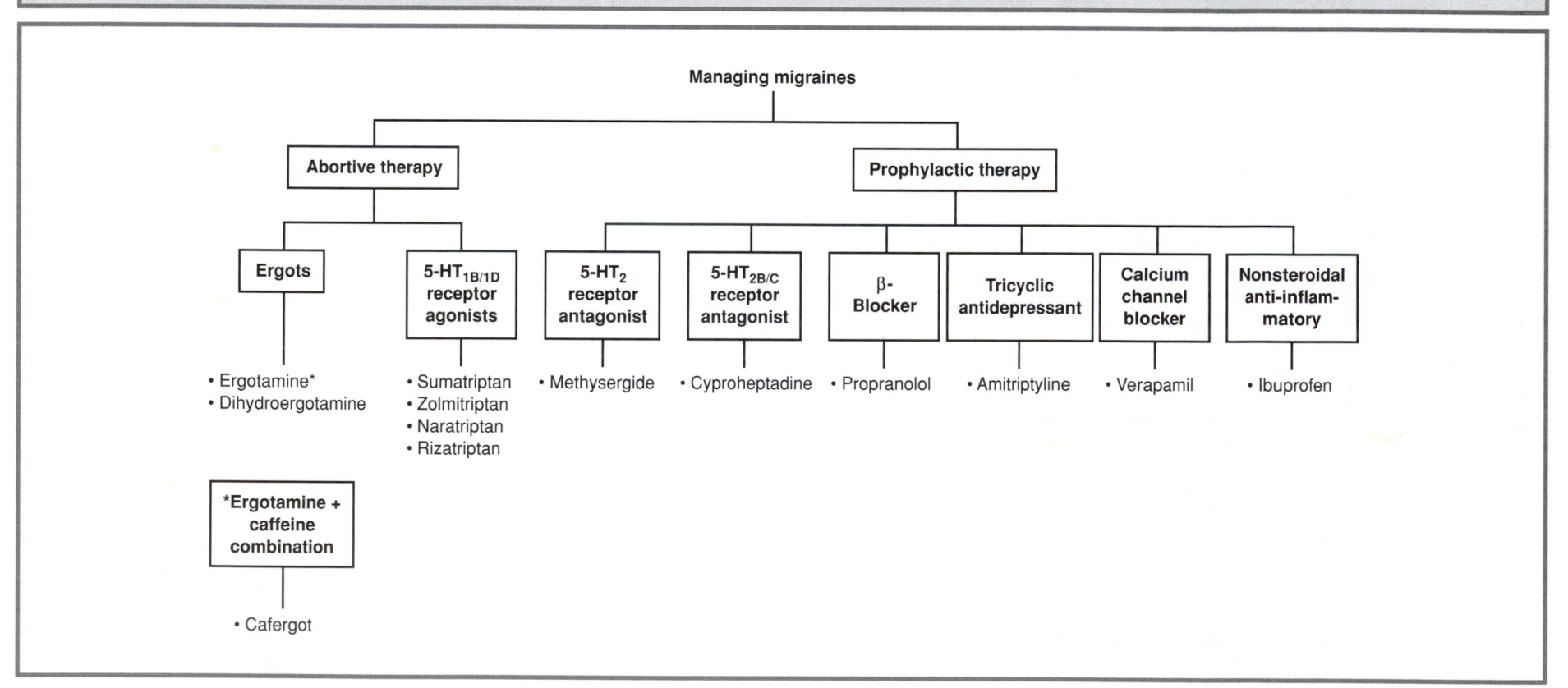

Drug	Pharmacokinetics	Mechanism of Action	Clinical Uses	Drawbacks and Side Effects
Ergots				
Ergotamine (Ergostat)	• **A:** Sublingual, PO, or rectal • **M:** Hepatic metabolism • **E:** Majority of metabolites excreted in bile	• 5-$HT_{1B/1D}$ receptor agonists • Thought that stimulation of these receptors causes vasoconstriction of intracranial vessels and inhibits release of peptides involved in sterile neurogenic inflammatory response from the sensory processes of the trigeminal nerve	• Abortive antimigraine medications • Best used at the onset of the headache • Almost always administered with caffeine	• Ergotism • GI problems (nausea, vomiting, diarrhea) • Uterine contractions • Cannot be used in patients with angina or other coronary vascular disease • "Dirty drugs" that act at a number of adrenergic and serotonergic receptors
Dihydro-ergotamine (DHE-45, Migranal)	• **A:** IM, IV, or intranasal • **M:** Hepatic metabolism • **E:** Majority of parent drug and metabolites excreted in urine; remainder in bile			
Caffeine and Ergotamine				
Ergotamine and caffeine (Cafergot)	• **A:** PO or rectal; caffeine seems to help ergotamine absorption • **M:** Hepatic metabolism • **E:** Majority of metabolites excreted in bile and urine			

Continued

ABORTIVE ANTIMIGRAINE THERAPY (Continued)

Drug	Pharmacokinetics	Mechanism of Action	Clinical Uses	Drawbacks and Side Effects
5-HT$_{1B/1D}$ Receptor Agonists				
Sumatriptan (Imitrex)	• **A:** SC, PO, or intranasal; poorly absorbed • **M:** Hepatic metabolism to inactive metabolite • **E:** Metabolite excreted in urine		• Abortive antimigraine therapy • Very high and selective affinity for 1D$_\alpha$, 1D$_\beta$, and 1F receptors with little affinity for other 5-HT or monoamine receptors • Do not produce ergotism • No GI upset (as seen with ergots)	• Limit dose of agents metabolized by MAO-A in patients taking MAO inhibitors • Cannot be used in patients with angina or other coronary vascular disease • Paresthesias • Warm/cold sensations • Neck/throat/jaw/chest pain/tightness/pressure • Nausea • Dizziness • Sleepiness
Zolmitriptan (Zomig)	• **A:** PO; well absorbed • **M:** Metabolized by hepatic P450 enzymes to inactive and active metabolites • **E:** Parent drug and metabolites excreted in urine and feces			
Naratriptan (Amerge)	• **A:** PO; well absorbed • **M:** Hepatic P450 metabolism to inactive metabolites • **E:** Parent drug and metabolites excreted in urine			
Rizatriptan (Maxalt)	• **A:** PO; complete absorption • **M:** Metabolized by MAO-A to inactive metabolite (minor amount of active metabolite formed) • **E:** Majority of parent drug and metabolites excreted in urine; remainder in feces			

Drug	Class	Pharmacokinetics	Mechanism of Action	Clinical Uses	Side Effects
Methysergide (Sansert)	• 5-HT$_2$ Receptor antagonist	• **A:** PO • **M:** Hepatic metabolism • **E:** Parent drug and metabolite excreted in urine	• Unknown; thought to produce therapeutic results via action on serotonin	• Prophylactic antimigraine therapy	• Fibrotic reactions • Leg muscle cramps • Fatigue • Nausea
Cyproheptadine (Periactin)	• 5-HT$_{2B/C}$ Receptor antagonists	• **A:** PO • **M:** Hepatic metabolism • **E:** Metabolites excreted in urine; metabolites and parent drug excreted in feces			• Nausea • Drowsiness • Weight gain
Propranolol (Inderal)	• β-Blocker	• **A:** PO and IV; well absorbed • **M:** Hepatic metabolism • **E:** Metabolites excreted in urine	• 5-HT$_{2B/C}$ receptor antagonist in doses employed • As methysergide and cyproheptadine		• Bronchoconstriction • Hypotension • Bradycardia • Sexual dysfunction
Amitriptyline (Elavil)	• TCA	• **A:** IM and PO; incompletely absorbed from the GI tract • **M:** Hepatic metabolism • **E:** Metabolites excreted in urine	• Possesses some 5-HT$_2$ blocking properties • As methysergide and cyproheptadine		• Cardiotoxicity including quinidine-like cardiac conduction block • Anticholinergic side effects • Hypotension due to α_1-blockade • Sexual dysfunction • Sedation

Continued

PROPHYLACTIC ANTIMIGRAINE THERAPY (Continued)

Drug	Class	Pharmacokinetics	Mechanism of Action	Clinical Uses	Side Effects
Verapamil (Calan)	• Calcium channel blocker	• **A:** PO; well absorbed • **M:** Hepatic metabolism • **E:** Majority of metabolites excreted in urine; remainder in feces	• May act by reducing synthesis of prostacyclin or by interfering with 5-HT mediated release of endothelial NO		• Constipation • Dizziness • Elevated LFTs • Hypotension • May be harmful in patients with left-sided heart failure or conduction abnormalities
Ibuprofen (Advil, Motrin)	• Nonsteroidal anti-inflammatory	• **A:** PO; well absorbed • **M:** Hepatic metabolism • **E:** Metabolites excreted in urine	• Appears to act by inhibiting synthesis of prostaglandins including prostacyclin	• Prophylactic antimigraine therapy • Also effective in treating mild to moderate migraines	• Low toxicity • Gastritis

VII. Antispastic Drugs

MECHANISM OF ACTION OF ANTISPASTIC DRUGS

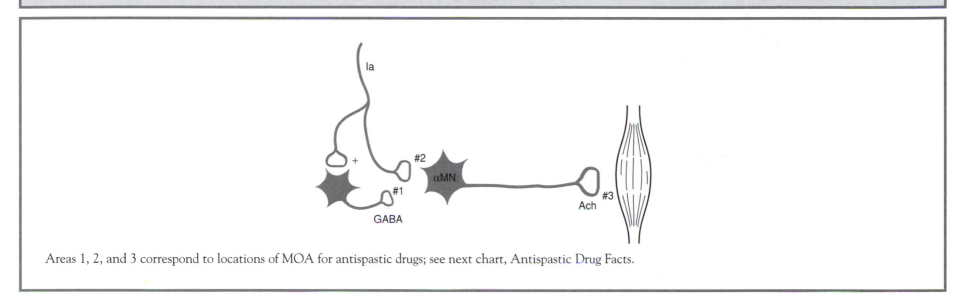

Areas 1, 2, and 3 correspond to locations of MOA for antispastic drugs; see next chart, Antispastic Drug Facts.

ANTISPASTIC DRUG FACTS

Drug	Pharmacokinetics	Mechanism of Action	Clinical Uses	Side Effects
Diazepam (Valium)	• **A:** IV and PO; good absorption • $t_{1/2}$: 20–80 hours • **M:** Hepatic metabolism to active metabolites • **E:** Active metabolites excreted in urine	• Positive allosteric modulation of $GABA_A$ • Acts at $GABA_A$ receptors on the terminal portion of the 1a axon • Acts at site #1 (see preceding chart Mechanism of Action of Antispastic Drugs)	• Spasticity associated with multiple sclerosis • Clonus and muscular rigidity in patients with spinal cord injuries	• Sedation • Respiratory depression • Physiologic dependence
Baclofen (Lioresal)	• **A:** Intrathecal and PO; rapidly absorbed from GI tract • $t_{1/2}$: 3–4 hours • **E:** Unchanged in urine	• Structural analog of GABA • $GABA_B$ agonist at terminal of 1a afferent neuron • Decreases release of excitatory amino acid neurotransmitter • May also decrease pain via inhibition of substance P release • Acts at site #2 (see preceding chart Mechanism of Action of Antispastic Drugs)	• Spasticity associated with multiple sclerosis • Clonus and muscular rigidity in patients with spinal cord injuries • Equal antispastic activity but less sedation than diazepam	• Sedation • Dizziness • Hypotension • Headache • Seizures • Weakness • Hallucinations and seizures upon abrupt withdrawal from PO administration
Tizanidine (Zanaflex)	• **A:** PO; absorbed rapidly and completely • $t_{1/2}$: 2.5 hours • **M:** Extensive first-pass hepatic metabolism to inactive metabolites • **E:** Metabolites excreted in both urine and feces	• Short acting α_2 and imidazoline agonist • Acts centrally to increase presynaptic inhibition of motor neurons • Decreases release of excitatory amino acid neurotransmitter at site #2 (see preceding chart Mechanism of Action of Antispastic Drugs)	• Spasticity associated with multiple sclerosis • Clonus and muscular rigidity in patients with spinal cord injuries	• Dry mouth • Sedation • Dizziness • Hypotension • Bradycardia

Drug	Pharmacokinetics	Mechanism of Action	Therapeutic Uses	Adverse Effects
Dantrolene (Dantrium)	• **A:** IV and PO; poorly absorbed from GI tract • $t_{1/2}$: 8 hours • **M:** Hepatic metabolism • **E:** Parent drug and metabolites excreted in urine	• Peripherally acting antispastic agent • Interferes with release of calcium from sarcoplasmic reticulum • Acts at site #3 (see preceding chart Mechanism of Action of Antispastic Drugs)	• Malignant hyperthermia	• General muscle weakness • Sedation • Hepatitis
Gabapentin (Neurontin)	• **A:** PO • $t_{1/2}$: 5–7 hours • **E:** Unchanged in urine	• Enhances the release of GABA via an unknown mechanism	• Spasticity associated with multiple sclerosis • Psychiatric disorders • Chronic pain • Epilepsy	• Dizziness • Sedation • Ataxia • Fatigue
Botulinum toxin (BoTox)	• **A:** IM • **D:** Does not enter systemic circulation in measurable quantities	• Enters motor neuron nerve terminal and inhibits release of Ach	• Local antispastic in disorders such as cerebral palsy, cervical dystonia, blepharospasm, and strabismus • Cosmetic treatment of wrinkles	• Weakness (eg, dysphagia in patients treated for cervical dystonia)

VIII. Local Anesthetics and Adjunctive Drugs

LOCAL ANESTHETICS AND ADJUNCTIVE DRUGS: SUMMARY TABLE

Pharmacokinetics		Mechanism of Action	Adverse Effects
Potency	**Dosing**		
• Measure of lipid solubility (ability to penetrate a hydrophobic environment) • Expressed as multiple of potency of procaine • Decreased pH decreases potency due to the inability of the cation to reach the site of action	• Maximum tolerated dose increased with slow administration or coadministration with vasoconstrictors (decrease drug removal by blood) or sedative/hypnotic drugs (increase seizure threshold) • Maximum tolerated dose decreased with hepatic disease • Maximum tolerated dose varies with drug	• Smaller, unmyelinated neurons are preferentially blocked by local anesthetics (ie, pain fibers) • As neuronal size and myelination increase, the effect decreases	• CNS: Circumoral numbness, tongue paresthesia, dizziness, tinnitus, diplopia, sedation, seizures (avoid IV injection) • CV: Decreased automaticity, contractility, and HR • Immunologic: Allergic reaction to PABA metabolite of choline esters

CLASSIFICATION OF LOCAL ANESTHETICS AND ADJUNCTIVE DRUGS

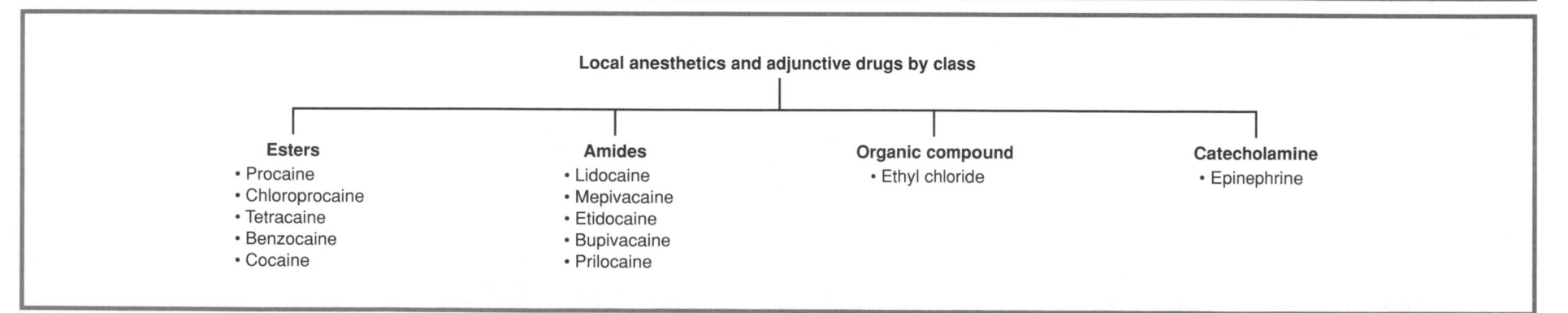

Local anesthetics and adjunctive drugs by class

Esters
- Procaine
- Chloroprocaine
- Tetracaine
- Benzocaine
- Cocaine

Amides
- Lidocaine
- Mepivacaine
- Etidocaine
- Bupivacaine
- Prilocaine

Organic compound
- Ethyl chloride

Catecholamine
- Epinephrine

LOCAL ANESTHETICS AND ADJUNCTIVE AGENTS: ESTERS

Drug	Potency	Pharmacokinetics	Mechanism of Action	Clinical Uses	Side Effects
Procaine (Novacaine)	1	• **B:** Low • **DOA:** Short • **OOA:** Slow • **M:** Rapid hydrolysis in plasma by plasma esterase; metabolites include PABA • **E:** Water soluble metabolites excreted in urine	• Block voltage-activated Na^+ channels from intracellular position • Produces reversible blockade of peripheral nerve conduction • Sympathetic blockade from neuraxis block	• Spinal anesthesia (mixed with tetracaine in obstetrics) • Local infiltration • Peripheral nerve block	• Low toxicity • Vasodilation
Chloroprocaine (Nesacaine)	4	• **B:** Low • **DOA:** Short • **OOA:** Rapid • **M:** Rapid hydrolysis in plasma by plasma esterase; metabolites include PABA • **E:** Water soluble metabolites excreted in urine		• Local infiltration • Epidural • Peripheral nerve block	
Tetracaine (Pontocaine)	16	• **B:** High • **DOA:** Long • **OOA:** Slow • **M:** Rapid hydrolysis in plasma by plasma esterase; metabolites include PABA • **E:** Water soluble metabolites excreted in urine		• Topical • Spinal • Peripheral nerve block	• Vasodilation

Continued

LOCAL ANESTHETICS AND ADJUNCTIVE AGENTS: ESTERS (Continued)

Drug	Potency	Pharmacokinetics	Mechanism of Action	Clinical Uses	Side Effects
Benzocaine (Americaine)	N/A	• **DOA:** Short • **OOA:** Slow • **M:** Metabolized by plasma esterase	• Accumulates within phospholipid cell membrane and deforms Na^+ channel resulting in decreased Na^+ conductance	• Topical sprays, creams, otic drops, sunburn and teething preparations	• Moderate toxicity • Methemoglobinemia possible with pediatric use
Cocaine	N/A	• **B:** Intermediate • **DOA:** Short • **OOA:** Slow • **M:** Metabolized in liver and plasma • **E:** Parent drug and metabolites excreted in urine	• MOA as a local anesthetic similar to procaine • Blocks reuptake of NE, DA, and 5-HT at nerve synapse	• Topical	• Vasoconstriction • CNS stimulation • Hypertension • Tachycardia • Arrhythmias

LOCAL ANESTHETICS AND ADJUNCTIVE AGENTS: AMIDES AND OTHER NONESTERS

Drug	Potency	Pharmacokinetics	Mechanism of Action	Clinical Uses	Side Effects
Amide					
Lidocaine (Xylocaine)	4	• **B:** High • **DOA:** Intermediate • **OOA:** Rapid • **M:** Hepatic microsomal enzymes	• Blocks voltage activated Na⁺ channels intracellularly • Produces reversible blockade of peripheral nerve conduction	• Topical creams and sprays • Local infiltration • Epidural • Spinal • Peripheral nerve block	• Moderate toxicity
Mepivacaine (Carbocaine)	2	• **B:** High • **DOA:** Intermediate • **OOA:** Rapid • **M:** Hepatic microsomal enzymes		• Local infiltration • Epidural • Peripheral nerve block	
Etidocaine (Duranest)	16	• **B:** High • **DOA:** Long • **OOA:** Rapid • **M:** Hepatic microsomal enzymes			
Bupivacaine (Marcaine)		• **B:** High • **DOA:** Long • **OOA:** Slow • **M:** Hepatic microsomal enzymes		• Local infiltration • Epidural (intense analgesia with minimal motor block) • Spinal • Peripheral nerve block	• Treatment-resistant ventricular arrhythmias • Cardiovascular collapse

Continued

LOCAL ANESTHETICS AND ADJUNCTIVE AGENTS: AMIDES AND OTHER NONESTERS (Continued)

Drug	Potency	Pharmacokinetics	Mechanism of Action	Clinical Uses	Side Effects
Prilocaine (Citanest)	3	• **B:** Intermediate • **DOA:** Intermediate • **OOA:** Rapid • **M:** Hepatic and renal metabolism		• Local infiltration (dental surgery) • Epidural • Peripheral nerve block	• Very low toxicity • Methemoglobinemia
Organic Compound					
Ethyl chloride	N/A	• **DOA:** Short • **OOA:** Rapid	Volatile liquid anesthetizes via rapid cooling during evaporation	• Topical anesthesia for minor surgery, injections, and dermatologic procedures • Treatment of myofascial pain • Anesthesia in nonclinical setting (athletic events)	• Flammable • Alteration of skin pigmentation following application • Hypersensitivity • Renal and hepatic toxicity prevent LTU
Catecholamine (Adrenergic Agonist)					
Epinephrine	N/A	• **DOA:** Intermediate • **OOA:** Rapid • **M:** Enzymatic degradation in liver and kidneys	• Vasoconstriction • Mixed with local anesthetics to prolong duration of action of drug	Reduces blood flow to anesthetized area to decrease removal of local anesthetic	• Toxicity from systemic absorption • Increased HR, BP, cardiac output • Decreased renal blood flow

IX. General Anesthetic Drugs

CLASSIFICATION OF GENERAL ANESTHETIC DRUGS

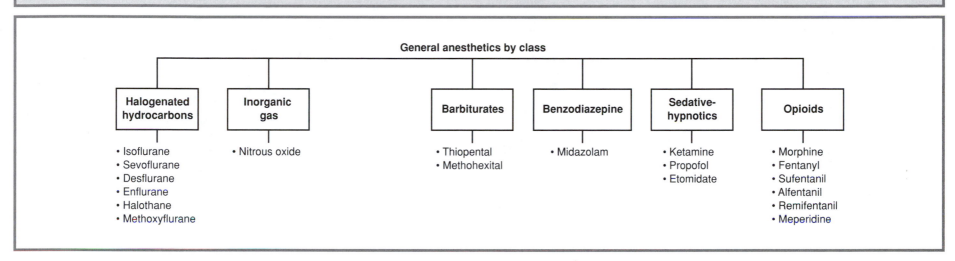

General anesthetics by class

Halogenated hydrocarbons
- Isoflurane
- Sevoflurane
- Desflurane
- Enflurane
- Halothane
- Methoxyflurane

Inorganic gas
- Nitrous oxide

Barbiturates
- Thiopental
- Methohexital

Benzodiazepine
- Midazolam

Sedative-hypnotics
- Ketamine
- Propofol
- Etomidate

Opioids
- Morphine
- Fentanyl
- Sufentanil
- Alfentanil
- Remifentanil
- Meperidine

GENERAL ANESTHETIC DRUGS: INHALED

Drug	MAC	B/G	Pharmacokinetics*	Clinical Uses	Side Effects
Halogenated Hydrocarbons					
☞ "Halogenated Hydrocarbons are inHaled as a vapor and eliminated via exHalation" "All increase ICP and decrease BP"					
Isoflurane (Forane)	1.15%	1.4	• **A:** Inhaled as a vapor • **M:** Minimal metabolism to fluoride • **E:** Via exhalation	• Bronchodilator • Depth of anesthesia can be rapidly adjusted • Cardiac output sustained • Arrhythmias uncommon • Potentiates action of skeletal muscle relaxants	• Pungent • Increases ICP • Increases HR • Decreases BP
Sevoflurane (Ultane)	1.7%	0.69	• **A:** Inhaled as a vapor • **M:** Small amount metabolized to fluoride • **E:** Via exhalation	• Bronchodilator • Low pungency, least irritating • Good for induction • Potentiates action of skeletal muscle relaxants	• Increases ICP • Decreases BP • Decreases ventilation
Desflurane (Suprane)	6%	0.42	• **A:** Inhaled; high vapor pressure requires special vaporizer • **M:** Minimal metabolism to fluoride • **E:** Via exhalation	• Very rapid induction and recovery • Potentiates action of skeletal muscle relaxants	• Pungent • Increases ICP • Decreases BP • Increases HR

Enflurane (Ethrane)	1.68%	1.9	• **A:** Inhaled as a vapor • **M:** Low peak levels of serum fluoride after metabolism but unlikely nephrotoxic • **E:** Via exhalation	• Smooth adjustments of depth of anesthesia are possible • Adequate skeletal muscle relaxant	• Pungent • Decreases ventilation • Increases ICP • Decreases BP • Avoid in patients with seizures or renal disease
Halothane (Fluothane)	0.74%	2.4	• **A:** Inhaled as a vapor • **M:** 20–25% oxidized in liver and kidney to trifluoroacetic acid • **E:** Via exhalation	• Low pungency • Bronchodilator • Minimal postoperative nausea and vomiting	• Increases ICP • Decreases ventilation • Decreases BP • Hepatotoxicity and fulminant hepatitis rare
Methoxyflurane (Penthrane)	0.16%	15.0	• **A:** Inhaled as a vapor • **M:** Significant metabolism to nephrotoxic metabolites (vasopressin-resistant high output renal failure) • **E:** Via exhalation	• Bronchodilator • Limited usefulness • Serves as a model of nephrotoxicity	• Increases ICP • Increased HR • Decreased BP
Inorganic Gas					
Nitrous oxide	105%	0.47	• **A:** Inhaled as a gas at room temperature • **M:** Minimal metabolism • **E:** Via exhalation	• Nonflammable, nonirritating • Little toxicity • Does not increase ICP • Rapid onset, short duration, and rapid recovery • Used in combination with intravenous and other inhalation agents to decrease their requirements	• Insufficient to produce surgical anesthesia as a sole agent • No muscle relaxation • Avoid in patients with closed air cavities (intestinal obstruction, pneumothorax, air embolus)

GENERAL ANESTHETIC DRUGS: INTRAVENOUS NONOPIOIDS

Drug	Pharmacokinetics	Clinical Uses	Side Effects
Barbiturates			
Thiopental (Pentothal) Methohexital (Brevital)	• **A:** IV • **OOA:** Rapid • **DOA:** Ultra-short • **M:** Hepatic • **E:** Renal	• Rapid recovery • Used during induction	• Irritating to vein • No analgesia • Possible hyperalgesia at subanesthetic doses • Peripheral vasodilation • Respiratory depression • Thiopental should be avoided in patients with abnormalities in porphyrin metabolism
Benzodiazepines			
Midazolam (Versed)	• **A:** IV, IM, PO • **OOA:** Rapid • **DOA:** Short • **M:** Hepatic • **E:** Renal	• 100% reversible with antagonist (flumazenil) • Anterograde amnesia • Preoperative anxiolysis; adjunct to local/regional/general anesthesia • ICU sedation	• Dose-related dependence • Drug interactions due to P450 metabolism • Possible CV depression • Does not reach complete surgical anesthesia as a sole agent
Sedative/Hypnotics			
Ketamine (Ketalar)	• **A:** IV, IM • **OOA:** Rapid • **DOA:** Short • **M:** Hepatic • **E:** Renal	• Produces dissociative anesthesia • No loss of consciousness • Rapid recovery • Low doses provide analgesia • Airway patency maintained • Used in short surgeries and painful procedures, especially in pediatrics	• CV stimulation • Increases ICP • Diplopia • Nystagmus • Emergence reactions (agitation)

Propofol (Diprivan)	• **A:** IV • **OOA:** Rapid • **DOA:** Short • **M:** Hepatic • **E:** Renal	• Used for induction • Maintenance of anesthesia during short cases • ICU sedation • Antiemetic properties	• Contraindicated in patients with egg allergy • Requires metabolism to end effect following long infusions or high doses • Irritating to vein • Decreases ventilation • Decreases BP • Decreases ICP • Not for use in children
Etomidate (Amidate)	• **A:** IV • **OOA:** Rapid • **DOA:** Short • **M:** Hepatic • **E:** Renal	• Used for induction • Supplement during maintenance • Rapid recovery	• Decreases cortisol levels (unresponsive to ACTH) • Decreases ICP • Nausea and vomiting

GENERAL ANESTHETIC DRUGS: INTRAVENOUS OPIOIDS

Drug	Pharmacokinetics	Clinical Uses	Drawbacks and Side Effects
Morphine (Duramorph)	• **A:** IV, IM, SC, PO • **OOA:** Intermediate • **DOA:** Intermediate • **M:** Hepatic • **E:** Renal	• Reduce dysphoria associated with pain • Increase pain tolerance • Reduce amount of other anesthetic agent when administered simultaneously • Used in patient-controlled analgesia, preoperative anxiolysis/analgesia/sedation, adjuncts to other anesthetics, and regional anesthesia • Minimal cardiovascular depression	• Histamine release • Nausea and vomiting • Respiratory depression • Decreased cough reflex • Venodilation (decreased BP) • Constipation
Fentanyl (Sublimaze)	• **A:** IV, IM, transdermal, PO • **OOA:** Rapid • **DOA:** Intermediate • **M:** Hepatic • **E:** Renal		
Sufentanil (Sufenta)	• **A:** IV • **OOA:** Immediate • **DOA:** Short • **M:** Hepatic • **E:** Renal	• More potent than fentanyl • Adjunct or primary anesthetic • Mixed with bupivacaine in epidural • Rapid recovery	• Respiratory depression • Constipation
Alfentanil (Alfenta)	• **A:** IV • **OOA:** Immediate • **DOA:** Short • **M:** Hepatic • **E:** Renal	• Adjunct or primary anesthetic • Rapid recovery	

Remifentanil (Ultiva)	• **A:** IV • **OOA:** Immediate • **DOA:** Short • **M:** Plasma/tissue esterases • **E:** Renal	• Adjunct or primary anesthetic • Rapid recovery	• Respiratory depression • Hypotension • Constipation
Meperidine (Demerol)	• **A:** IV, IM • **OOA:** Intermediate • **DOA:** Intermediate • **M:** Hepatic • **E:** Renal	• Adjunct to other anesthetic • Obstetric anesthesia • Preoperative and short-term IV pain control	• Toxic metabolites • Weak agent • Decreases BP • Decreases ventilation • Decreases cough reflex • Constipation

☞ **OP**ioids **OPp**RES**s** **RES**piration

"…t**ANILS**"
Administration: IV;
Excretion: re**N**al; **I**mmediate action; **L**asts a **S**hort time

FOUR COMPONENTS, FOUR STAGES, AND FOUR KEYS TO ANESTHESIA

Components of Good Anesthesia	1. Loss of consciousness and amnesia: patient does not respond to command and will have no recall of surgical procedures; produced by nitrous oxide, benzodiazepines, or very low doses of any general anesthetic 2. Analgesia: elimination of the sensation of pain; produced by IV narcotic analgesics 3. Blunting of protective reflexes: primarily blunting of protective airway reflexes; produced by general anesthetics 4. Muscle relaxation: reduction in the resting muscle tone; produced by muscle relaxants
Stages of Anesthesia	1. Analgesia (buzz): produced by nitrous oxide or ketamine, patient remains conscious 2. Excitement (spazz): deeper level of analgesia during which the patient is unresponsive, but because the cortex is depressed, there is disinhibition of activity and the patient flails 3. Surgical anesthesia (out): blunts protective reflexes, provides amnesia, eliminates sensation of pain, creates a still and bloodless field for surgeon 4. Medullary depression (death): cardiovascular and respiratory centers cease to function leading to death
Keys to Anesthesia	1. Maintain homeostasis: oxygenation and ventilation 2. Protection of the patient from injury 3. Provide a bloodless field (via vasoconstriction provided by adjuncts such as epinephrine) 4. Optimize patient's medical condition before and after surgery

NONANESTHETIC DRUGS USED DURING GENERAL ANESTHESIA

Class	Example	Clinical Use	Side Effects
Sedatives	• Benzodiazepines (eg, midazolam)	• Sedation	• Decrease pain tolerance
Muscle relaxants	• Depolarizing (eg, succinylcholine) and nondepolarizing (eg, pancuronium)	• Prevent movement during procedures • Causes muscular relaxation, easing surgical access	• No analgesia or amnesia

X. Neuromuscular Blockers

NEUROMUSCULAR BLOCKERS: SUMMARY TABLE

Class	Pharmacokinetics				Mechanism of Action	Clinical Uses
☞ NM blockers ending in "Onium" are all sterOid derivatives; those ending in "Urium", "Urine" or "Uranine" are all isoqUinoline derivatives	**Administration**	**Onset of Action**	**Distribution**	**Metabolism**		
	IV	Important for determining appropriate time for intubation	All are ionized, therefore limited distribution occurs	Steroid derivatives must undergo hepatic biotransformation to achieve their active form	All NM blockers are nondepolarizing EXCEPT succinylcholine, which causes depolarization	Used by anesthesiologists in the OR for surgical muscular relaxation

NONDEPOLARIZING AND DEPOLARIZING NEUROMUSCULAR BLOCKERS

Drug	Class	Pharmacokinetics	Mechanism of Action	Side Effects
Nondepolarizing NM Blockers				
Tubocurarine	• Isoquinoline derivatives	• **DOA:** Long • **OOA:** Slow • **E:** Via kidney (some have minor hepatic elimination as well)	• Competitive inhibition of Ach at the nicotinic receptors of the NMJ	• Moderate histamine release • Hypotension (due to histamine release and ganglionic blockade)
Metocurine		• **DOA:** Long • **OOA:** Slow • **E:** Via kidney (some have minor hepatic elimination as well)		• Slight histamine release • Hypotension (due to histamine release and ganglionic blockade)

Continued

NONDEPOLARIZING AND DEPOLARIZING NEUROMUSCULAR BLOCKERS (Continued)

Drug	Class	Pharmacokinetics	Mechanism of Action	Side Effects
Doxacurium		• **DOA:** Long • **OOA:** Slow • **E:** Via kidney		• Low incidence of toxicity
Mivacurium		• **DOA:** Short • **OOA:** Rapid • **M:** Via plasma cholinesterase		• Slight histamine release • Hypotension (due histamine release and ganglionic blockade)
Cisatracurium		• **DOA:** Intermediate • **OOA:** Intermediate • **M:** Spontaneous breakdown		• Low incidence of toxicity
Atracurium		• **DOA:** Intermediate • **OOA:** Intermediate • **M:** Spontaneous breakdown, plasma cholinesterase and hepatic metabolism (minor)		• Major metabolite (laudanosine) has long $t_{1/2}$, crosses BBB and may cause seizures • Slight histamine release • Hypotension (due to histamine release and ganglionic blockade)
Pancuronium	• Steroid derivatives	• **DOA:** Long • **OOA:** Slow • **E:** Via kidney		• Moderate blockade of cardiac muscarinic receptors causing tachycardia • Blocks autonomic ganglia
Pipecuronium		• **DOA:** Long • **OOA:** Slow • **E:** Via kidney		• Low incidence of toxicity

Vecuronium		• **DOA:** Intermediate • **OOA:** Intermediate • **M:** Hepatic • **E:** Biliary	• Low incidence of toxicity
Rocuronium		• **DOA:** Intermediate • **OOA:** Rapid • **M:** Hepatic • **E:** Biliary	• Low incidence of toxicity
Rapacuronium		• **DOA:** Short • **OOA:** Rapid • **E:** Hepatic	• Large blockade of cardiac muscarinic receptors causing tachycardia
Gallamine	• Substituted ammonium salt	• **DOA:** Long • **OOA:** Slow • **E:** Via kidney (some have minor hepatic elimination as well)	• No longer marketed in the United States • Large blockade of cardiac muscarinic receptors causing tachycardia
Depolarizing NM Blocker			
Succinylcholine	• Dimer of acetylcholine	• **DOA:** Short • **OOA:** Rapid • **M:** Via plasma cholinesterase	• Acts like a nicotinic agonist at NMJ • Causes fasciculations followed by paralysis due to persistent depolarization of the end plate	• Hyperkalemia (especially in patients with muscular dystrophy, peripheral nerve dysfunction, burn or spinal cord injury) • Increased intraocular pressure • Increased intragastric pressure (emesis) • Muscle pain/damage • Slight histamine release • Stimulates autonomic ganglia • Stimulates cardiac muscarinic receptors causing bradycardia • Interactions with other medications (eg, aminoglycosides)

CHAPTER 6

MEDICATIONS AFFECTING CARDIAC AND RENAL FUNCTION

VI. DIURETICS

Classification of Diuretics

Thiazide, Loop, and
Potassium-sparing Diuretics

Carbonic Acid Inhibitor and
Osmotic Diuretics

Serum Electrolyte Effects
of Diuretics

VII. ANTIHYPER-
LIPIDEMIC DRUGS

Classification of
Antihyperlipidemic Drugs

Antihyperlipidemics: Bile
Acid Sequestrants and
Nicotinic Acid

Antihyperlipidemics:
HMG-CoA Reductase
Inhibitors

Antihyperlipidemic: Fibric
Acid Derivatives

Summary of
Antihyperlipidemic Drug
Effects

Effects of
Antihyperlipidemics
on Lipoproteins

VIII. MANAGING
COAGULOPATHY

Drugs Used in Clotting
Disorders

Drugs Used to Reduce
Clotting: Anticoagulants,
Thrombolytics, and
Antiplatelets

Drugs Used to Facilitate
Clotting

Acanthosis Nigricans	Warty growths and hyperpigmentation characteristically found the in the axilla and groin; associated with certain drugs, endocrine disorders, obesity, or malignancy.
Alopecia	Absence or loss of hair.
Angina	Chest discomfort caused by insufficient cardiac blood flow resulting in cardiac ischemia.
Conn's Syndrome	Primary hyperaldosteronism.
Hypertrichosis	Excessive hair growth.
Lupus-Like Syndrome	Drug-induced syndrome resembling the symptoms associated with SLE; rarely demonstrates nephritic component.
Pheochromocytoma	Catecholamine-secreting tumor of the adrenal gland.
Quinidine Syncope	Recurrent light-headedness and fainting associated with use of quinidine.
Rhabdomyolysis	Destruction of skeletal muscle cells.
Thrombotic Thrombocytopenic Purpura	Coagulopathy seen in adults; associated with central nervous system involvement.
Tinnitis	Ringing in the ears.
Tolerance	Repeated administration of medication leads to decreased effectiveness.
Torsades de Pointes	A ventricular arrhythmia often induced by antiarrhythmic drugs (especially those that prolong the QT interval). Its morphology is that of a polymorphic ventricular tachycardia often with an increasing then decreasing QRS amplitude.
Wolff-Parkinson-White Syndrome	Syndrome associated with ventricular arrhythmias due to the presence of an accessory conduction pathway between the SA and AV nodes.

I. Antianginal Drugs

CLASSIFICATION OF ANTIANGINAL DRUGS

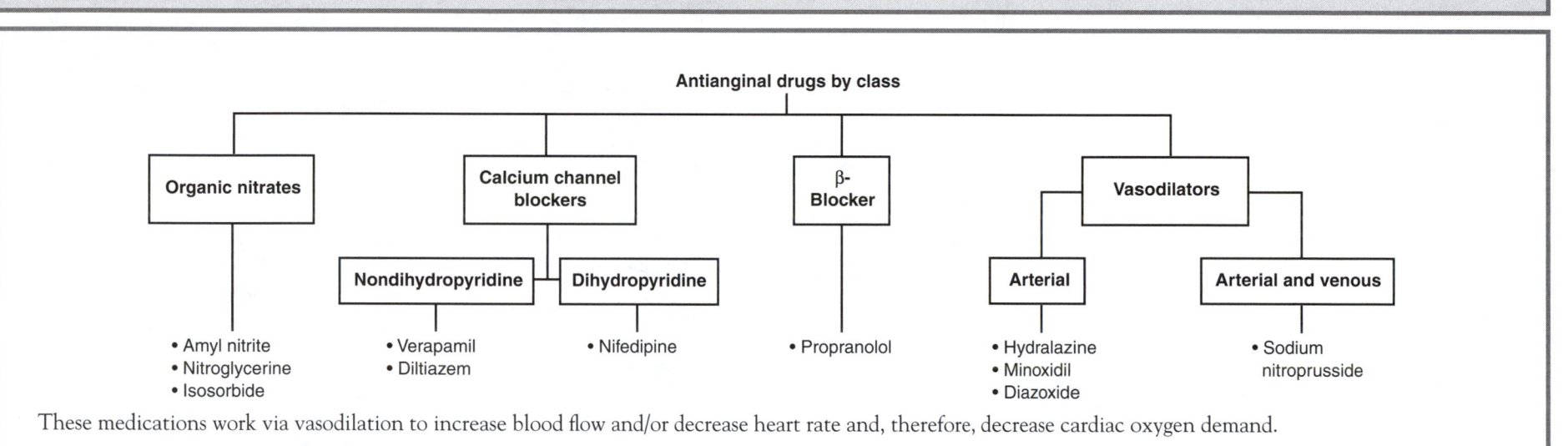

These medications work via vasodilation to increase blood flow and/or decrease heart rate and, therefore, decrease cardiac oxygen demand.

ANTIANGINALS: ORGANIC NITRATES, CALCIUM CHANNEL BLOCKERS, AND β-BLOCKER

Drug	Pharmacokinetics	Mechanism of Action	Clinical Uses	Side Effects
Organic Nitrates				
Amyl nitrite (Aspirols, Vaporole)	• **A:** Inhalation of volatile substance • **M:** Rapidly metabolized • **E:** One third excreted unchanged in urine	• Converted to nitric oxide intracellularly, which activates guanylate cyclase, leading to the following cascade of events: – an increase in cGMP – dephosphorylation of myosin light chain – relaxation of vascular smooth muscle – vasodilation • Venous dilation decreases preload • Vasodilation increases blood flow to myocardium	• Acute stable and unstable angina (short-acting nitrates) • Angina prophylaxis (longer-acting nitrates, eg, isosorbide dinitrate)	• Headache • Tolerance • Large degree of cross tolerance between organic nitrates • Systemic compensation (salt and water retention) may also be involved in loss of effectiveness
Nitroglycerin (Nitro-Bid, Nitro-Dur)	• **A:** Sublingual, PO, IV, ointment, or patches • **M:** Hepatic metabolism to active metabolites		• Acute stable and unstable angina (short-acting nitrates) • Angina prophylaxis (longer-acting nitrates, eg, isosorbide dinitrate) • Hypertension	
Isosorbide dinitrate (Isordil, Sorbitrate)	• **A:** Sublingual, PO, IV, ointment, or patches • **M:** Hepatic metabolism to active metabolites • **E:** Metabolites excreted in urine		• Acute stable and unstable angina (short-acting nitrates) • Angina prophylaxis (longer-acting nitrates, eg, isosorbide dinitrate) • CHF	

Continued

ANTIANGINALS: ORGANIC NITRATES, CALCIUM CHANNEL BLOCKERS, AND β-BLOCKER (Continued)

Drug	Pharmacokinetics	Mechanism of Action	Clinical Uses	Side Effects
Non-Dihydropyridine Calcium Channel Blockers				
Verapamil (Calan, Isoptin)	• **A:** PO and IV • **M:** Extensive first-pass hepatic metabolism; metabolized by P450 enzymes to active metabolites • **E:** In urine and feces	• Reduce Ca^{2+} influx • Resulting reduction of IC Ca^{2+} leads to smooth muscle relaxation • Result in decreased myocardial contractile force and decreased arterial tone and systemic vascular resistance	• Stable, unstable, and variant angina • Supraventricular arrhythmias • Ventricular rate control in atrial flutter and fibrillation • Hypertension	• Bradycardia • Constipation • Decreased cardiac contractility • Hypotension • Increases digoxin levels
Diltiazem (Cardizem, Dilacor)	• **A:** PO and IV • **M:** Extensive first-pass hepatic metabolism; metabolized by P450 enzymes to less active metabolites • **E:** In urine and feces		• Stable and variant angina • Supraventricular arrhythmias • Ventricular rate control in atrial flutter and fibrillation • Hypertension	• Bradycardia • Hypotension • Decreased cardiac contractility

Dihydropyridine Calcium Channel Blocker

Nifedipine (Adalat, Procardia)	• **A:** PO • **M:** Extensive first-pass hepatic metabolism; metabolized by P450 enzymes to inactive metabolites • **E:** In urine and feces		• Stable and variant angina • Hypertension	• Flushing • Headache • Hypotension (rapid decrease in BP can exacerbate ischemia) • Peripheral edema • Reflex tachycardia

β-Blocker

Propranolol (Inderal)	• **A:** PO and IV • **M:** Extensive first-pass hepatic metabolism • **E:** Parent drug and metabolites excreted in urine and feces	• Decreases heart rate and contractility to reduce oxygen demand of the heart • Increases time in diastole • Increases coronary blood flow • Increases exercise tolerance and duration • Decreases frequency and severity of angina attacks	• Stable and unstable angina • Often used in combination with nitrates or calcium channel blockers	• Contraindicated in patients with asthma, diabetes, PVD, or COPD • Combine carefully with verapamil and diltiazem because additive negative ionotropic effects lead to bradyarrhythmias

ANTIANGINALS: VASODILATORS

Drug	Pharmacokinetics	Mechanism of Action	Clinical Uses	Drawbacks and Side Effects
Arterial Vasodilators				
Hydralazine (Apresoline)	• **A:** PO, IM, and IV • **M:** Extensive first-pass hepatic metabolism; hepatic acetylation (remember that certain patient populations have varying rates of acetylation) • **E:** Metabolites excreted in urine	• Arterial smooth muscle relaxation and vasodilation (probably through action on cAMP and Ca^{2+})	• Angina • Hypertension • CHF	• Toxicity in slow acetylators • Tachycardia • Headache • Dizziness • Nausea • Sweating • Flushing • Nasal congestion • Lupus-like syndrome
Minoxidil (Loniten)	• **A:** PO and topical • **M:** Hepatic metabolism • **E:** Metabolites excreted in urine	• Inhibits PDE leading to increased levels of cAMP, which through Ca^{2+} modulation leads to arterial smooth muscle relaxation and vasodilation	• Angina • Hypertension • Alopecia	• Tachycardia • Massive fluid retention • Hypertrichosis • ECG changes • Pericarditis
Diazoxide (Proglycem)	• **A:** PO or IV • **M:** Partial hepatic metabolism • **E:** Parent drug and metabolites excreted in urine	• Decreases peripheral vascular resistance via direct vasodilatory effect on smooth muscle in peripheral arterioles	• Angina • Acute hypertensive emergencies • Hypoglycemia (secondary to hyperinsulinemia via inhibition of insulin release)	• Reflex tachycardia

Arterial and Venous Vasodilator

Sodium nitroprusside (Nitropress)	• **A:** IV • **M:** Local metabolism by tissues and erythrocytes • **E:** Metabolites excreted in urine, feces, and exhaled air	• Dilates arteries and veins	• Angina • Acute hypertensive emergencies • CHF	• By-product of metabolism is cyanide, which is metabolized in the liver by rhodanase to thiocyanate (water soluble and excreted in urine) • Cyanide poisoning in patients with poor diets (alcoholics), where it leads to decreased sulfur availability or when administered in high doses for long period of time • Drug is broken down by UV light so IV bag must be wrapped in foil

EFFECTS OF NITRATES COMBINED WITH β-BLOCKERS

β-Blockers and nitrates are often combined to achieve vasodilation and decreased contractility to relieve angina without causing an increase in HR (reflex tachycardia).

Drug Class	Heart Rate	Arterial Pressure	Contractility
Nitrates	↑	↓ (vasodilation)	↓ then ↑ (reflex tachycardia)
β-Blockers	↓ or ↔	↔	↓
β-Blockers and nitrates	↔	↓	↓ or ↔
☞ Think of this chart as summation vertically:	Heart rate of increase (nitrates) plus decrease (β-blockers) equals no effect (nitrates and β-blockers).	Arterial pressure of decrease plus no effect equals decrease.	Contractility of decrease then increase, plus decrease equals decrease or no effect.

↔, no effect.

MECHANISMS OF ACTION OF ANTIANGINAL DRUGS

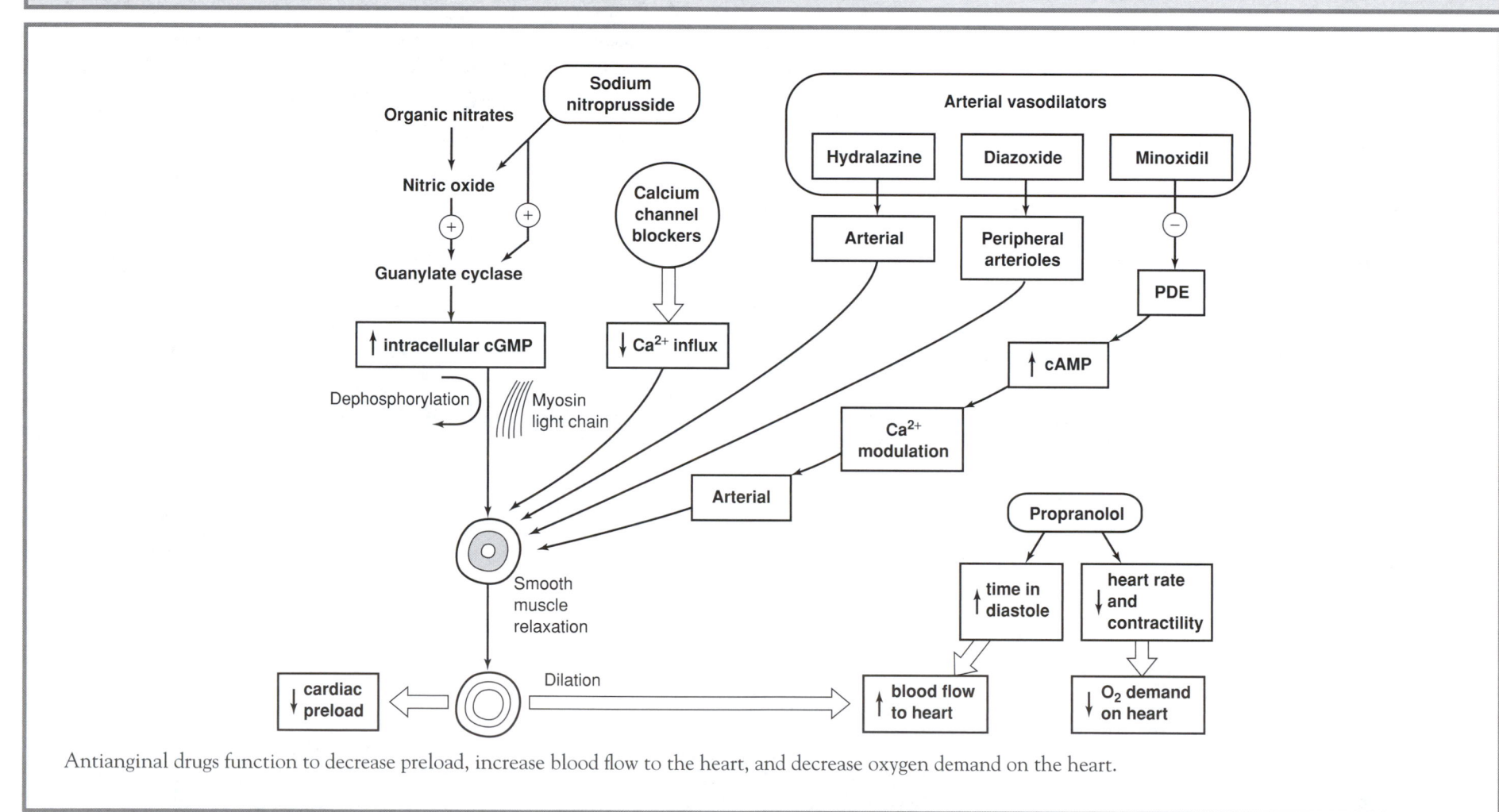

Antianginal drugs function to decrease preload, increase blood flow to the heart, and decrease oxygen demand on the heart.

II. Antiarrhythmics

CLASSIFICATION OF ANTIARRHYTHMIC DRUGS

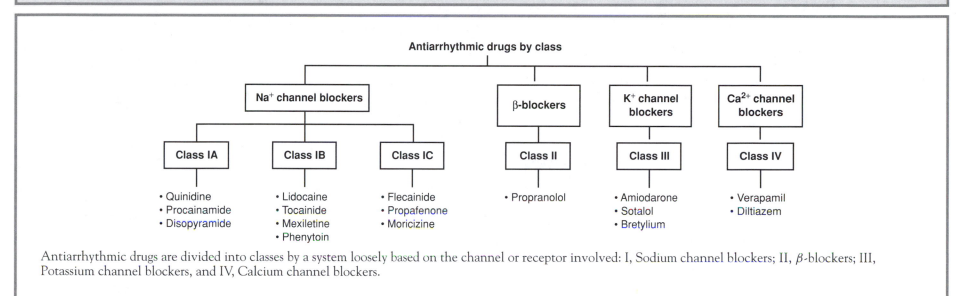

Antiarrhythmic drugs are divided into classes by a system loosely based on the channel or receptor involved: I, Sodium channel blockers; II, β-blockers; III, Potassium channel blockers, and IV, Calcium channel blockers.

Modified from Trevor AJ, Katzung BG, Masters SB: *Katzung & Trevor's Pharmacology Examination & Board Review*, 6th ed, p 120. Originally published by Appleton & Lange. © 2002 by the McGraw-Hill Companies, Inc.

CLASS I ANTIARRHYTHMICS

Drug	Pharmacokinetics	Mechanism of Action	Clinical Uses	Drawbacks and Side Effects
Class IA				
Quinidine (Quinaglute)	• **A:** PO and IV • **M:** Hepatic metabolism • **E:** Parent drug and metabolites excreted in urine	• Inhibit fast Na^+ channel by blocking activated Na^+ channels • Weakly block K^+ channels (reduces repolarization), which increases AP duration (manifests as a lengthening of QT interval)	• All type of arrhythmias • Especially useful for atrial flutter, atrial fibrillation, and ventricular tachycardia	• Antimuscarinic activity can suppress vagal tone leading to an increase in AV conduction, which may cause tachycardia and arrhythmias • Refractory heterogeneity: depressed conduction can further lead to torsades de pointes and eventual quinidine syncope • Chichonism • GI symptoms (nausea, vomiting, diarrhea) • Digitalis toxicity: quinidine increases plasma digoxin levels
Procainamide (Procanbid, Pronestyl)	• **A:** PO, IV, IM • **M:** Hepatic metabolism to N-acetylprocainamide (NAPA) • **E:** In urine		• Same as above • Especially useful for sustained ventricular arrhythmias associated with acute MI	• GI symptoms (nausea, vomiting) • Hypotension • LTU can lead to lupus-like syndrome via unknown mechanism • Torsades de pointes
Disopyramide (Norpace)	• **A:** PO • **M:** 50% hepatic metabolism • **E:** Parent drug and metabolites excreted in urine		• Ventricular arrhythmias	• Antimuscarinic activity can suppress vagal tone leading to an increase in AV conduction, which may cause tachycardia and arrhythmias • Negative inotropic effects may precipitate failure in patients with ventricular dysfunction • Antimuscarinic side effects • Torsades de pointes

Class IB

Lidocaine (Xylocaine)	• **A:** IV, IM • **M:** Hepatic metabolism • **E:** Parent drug and metabolites excreted in urine	• Inhibit both inactive and active Na$^+$ channels • Act preferentially on depolarized, arrhythmogenic tissue • Shorten AP duration	• Suppression of recurrent ventricular tachycardia and fibrillation	• CNS side effects (tremor, light-headedness, nausea of central origin, paresthesias)
Tocainide (Tonocard)	• **A:** PO • **E:** Unchanged in urine		• Ventricular arrhythmias	• GI side effects (nausea) • Neurologic side effects (tremor, lethargy, blurred vision)
Mexiletine (Mexitil)	• **A:** PO • **M:** 90% metabolized to inactive metabolites • **E:** Parent drug and metabolites excreted in urine			
Phenytoin (Dilantin)	• **A:** PO and IV • **M:** Partial hepatic metabolism • **E:** Parent drug and metabolites excreted in urine		• Ventricular tachycardia and paroxysmal atrial tachycardia	• Hypotension • Vertigo • Lethargy • Gingivitis • Lupus • Pulmonary infiltrates

Continued

CLASS I ANTIARRHYTHMICS (Continued)

Drug	Pharmacokinetics	Mechanism of Action	Clinical Uses	Drawbacks and Side Effects
Class IC				
Flecainide (Tambocor)	• **A:** PO and IV; well absorbed • **M:** Hepatic metabolism to inactive metabolites • **E:** Parent drug and metabolites excreted in urine	• Inhibit fast Na^+ channels • Especially effective in the His-Purkinje system (widens QRS complex) • Usually little effect on AP duration	• Ventricular arrhythmias • Supraventricular arrhythmias • Paroxysmal supraventricular tachycardia • Paroxysmal atrial fibrillation/flutter • Arrhythmias associated with Wolff-Parkinson-White syndrome	• Prolongation of QRS complex • Proarrhythmic • CNS side effects
Propafenone (Rythmol)	• **A:** PO and IV • **M:** Hepatic metabolism • **E:** Parent drug and metabolites mainly excreted in feces		• Supraventricular arrhythmias	• Metallic taste • Constipation • Prolongation of QRS interval • Proarrhythmia • GI side effects
Moricizine (Ethmozine)	• **A:** PO • **M:** Hepatic metabolism • **E:** Metabolites excreted in urine		• Ventricular arrhythmias	• Dizziness • Nausea

CLASSES II, III, AND IV ANTIARRHYTHMICS

Drug	Pharmacokinetics	Mechanism of Action	Clinical Uses	Side Effects
Class II				
β-Blockers	• **A:** IV or PO	• Block sympathetic effects on the heart • Affect primarily the SA and AV nodes • Decrease SA node automaticity and AV nodal conduction	• Supraventricular arrhythmia • Control of ventricular rate during atrial flutter and fibrillation	• Contraindicated in asthmatic patients (bronchoconstriction) • Sudden withdrawal can lead to rebound hypersensitivity
Class III				
Amiodarone (Cordarone)	• **A:** IV and PO; slow GI absorption; long period to reach steady state • **M:** Hepatic metabolism to active metabolite • **E:** Excreted by lacrimal glands, skin, and biliary tract	• Prolongs AP duration by blocking K$^+$ channels • Does not effect conduction velocity • Blocks Na$^+$ channels • Blocks calcium channels • Some β-blocker activity • Coronary and peripheral vasodilator	• Ventricular tachyarrhythmias (especially in post MI and CHF patients) • Atrial fibrillation/flutter • Paroxysmal supraventricular tachycardia • Arrhythmias associated with Wolff-Parkinson-White syndrome	• Pulmonary fibrosis • Hypothyroidism or hyperthyroidism • Paresthesias/tremor • Torsades de points
Sotalol (Betapace)	• **A:** PO; well absorbed • **E:** Unchanged in urine	• Prolongs AP duration • Possesses β-blocker and potassium-channel blocking activity		• Bradycardia • Bronchospasm • Fatigue • Torsades de points

Continued

CLASSES II, III, AND IV ANTIARRHYTHMICS (Continued)

Drug	Pharmacokinetics	Mechanism of Action	Clinical Uses	Side Effects
Bretylium (Bretylol)	• **A:** IM and IV • **E:** Unchanged in urine	• Same as amiodarone • Blocks the release of catecholamines from nerves after initial stimulation of release	• Ventricular arrhythmias (especially in post MI patients)	• Hypotension • Sympathomimetic effects
Class IV				
Verapamil (Calan, Isoptin)	• **A:** PO and IV • **M:** Extensive first-pass hepatic metabolism; metabolized by P450 enzymes to active metabolites • **E:** Metabolites excreted in urine and feces	• Calcium channel blocker that effects mainly the SA and AV nodes • Reduces SA node automaticity and AV nodal conduction	• Supraventricular arrhythmias • Ventricular rate control in atrial flutter and fibrillation	• Contraindicated with β-blockers • Bradycardia • Constipation • Decreased cardiac contractility • Hypotension • Lassitude • Nervousness • Peripheral edema
Diltiazem (Cardizem, Dilacor)	• **A:** PO and IV • **M:** Extensive first-pass hepatic metabolism; metabolized by P450 enzymes to less active metabolites • **E:** In urine and feces			• Bradycardia • Decreased cardiac contractility • Hypotension

III. Managing Congestive Heart Failure

CLASSIFICATION OF CHF DRUGS

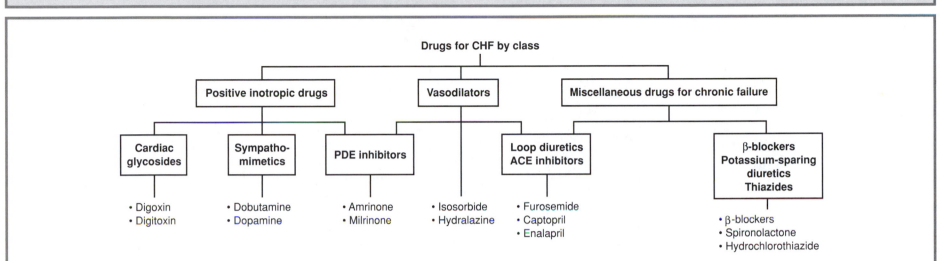

Steps in the treatment of CHF:

1. Reduce the workload of the heart (**ABC**): A) limit **A**ctivity level, B) **B**ring down [reduce] weight, C) **C**ontrol hypertension.

2. Restrict sodium.

3. Restrict water intake (rare).

4. Administer diuretics.

5. Administer ACE inhibitors and digitalis compounds.

6. Administer vasodilators.

CHF THERAPY: POSITIVE INOTROPIC DRUGS AND VASODILATORS

Drug	Pharmacokinetics	Mechanism of Action	Clinical Uses	Side Effects
Cardiac Glycosides				
Digoxin (Lanoxin, Lanoxicaps)	• **A:** IV or PO • **M:** Small amount metabolized in liver • **E:** Majority excreted unchanged in urine	• Inhibit the Na^+/K^+ ATPase, leading to an increase in IC Na^+ • Increase in IC Na^+ leads to a decrease in activity for the Na^+/Ca^{2+} exchanger, resulting in an increase in IC Ca^{2+}	• Treatment of chronic CHF • Therapeutic index is very low (high risk) • Digitalis compounds must be administered slowly and in small doses	**Cardiac side effects include:** • AV junctional rhythm • Premature ventricular depolarization • AV blockade **Noncardiac side effects include:**
Digitoxin (Digitaline)	• **A:** PO • **M:** Metabolized in liver • **E:** Metabolites excreted in bile	• Increase in IC Ca^{2+} means that the amount of Ca^{2+} present during an AP is higher, leading to a more forceful contraction • Direct electrical effects on the heart include decrease in AP duration, ectopic beats, and arrhythmias		• Nausea • Color vision abnormality • Anorexia • Diarrhea • Disorientation • Gynecomastia • Digoxin levels in plasma double when coadministered with quinidine • Hypokalemia can increase the risk of toxicity by worsening arrhythmia

Sympathomimetic

Dobutamine (Dobutrex)	• **A:** IV • **M:** Metabolized in urine and plasma by COMT • **E:** Metabolites excreted in urine	• Leads to an elevation of cAMP and subsequent positive inotropic effects • Low chronotropic activity	• Treatment of acute CHF	• Increased HR, BP • Angina
Dopamine (Intropin)	• **A:** IV • **M:** Metabolized in liver, kidneys, and plasma by MAO and COMT • **E:** Metabolites excreted in urine	• Causes release of NE at the heart, which leads to β-adrenergic stimulation • Stimulates β_1-receptors • Inhibits NE release in the periphery causing vasodilation	• Treatment of acute CHF • Also used to treat acute renal failure, shock, and cardiac arrest	• Dyspnea • Angina • Tachycardia • Headache • Nausea • Vomiting

PDE Inhibitors

Amrinone (Inocor)	• **A:** IV • **M:** Hepatic metabolism • **E:** Parent drug and metabolites excreted in urine and feces	• Inhibition of PDE leads to an elevation of cAMP • Selective for cardiac isoform of PDE • Bypass receptor so desensitization is avoided (LTU option is prevented by toxicity)	• Treatment of acute CHF	• Hepatotoxicity • Nausea and vomiting • Thrombocytopenia
Milrinone (Primacor)				• Less hepatotoxicity or bone marrow toxicity than amrinone

Continued

CHF THERAPY: POSITIVE INOTROPIC DRUGS AND VASODILATORS (Continued)

Drug	Pharmacokinetics	Mechanism of Action	Clinical Uses	Side Effects
Vasodilators				
Isosorbide dinitrate (Isordil, Sorbitrate)	• **A:** Sublingual, PO, IV, ointment, or patches • **M:** Hepatic metabolism to active metabolites • **E:** Metabolites excreted in urine	• Reduce the workload of the heart by reducing the afterload via arteriolar dilation and reducing the preload via venous dilation	• In patients with high filling pressures and pulmonary congestion • Angina prophylaxis	• Reflex tachycardia (prevented by use with β-blocker) • Tolerance • Cross tolerance • Headache
Hydralazine (Apresoline)	• **A:** PO, IM, and IV • **M:** Extensive first-pass hepatic metabolism; hepatic acetylation (remember that certain patient populations have varying rates of acetylation) • **E:** Metabolites excreted in urine		• In patients with low ventricular output, use an arteriolar dilator such as hydralazine • Hypertension • Angina	• Tachycardia • Headache • Dizziness • Nausea • Sweating • Flushing • Nasal congestion • Lupus-like syndrome

CHF THERAPY: DIURETICS AND ACE INHIBITORS

Drug	Pharmacokinetics	Mechanism of Action	Clinical Uses	Side Effects
Thiazide Diuretic				
Hydrochlorothiazide (HCTZ, HydroDIURIL)	• **A:** PO • **E:** Unchanged in urine	• Reduces salt and water retention, thereby reducing ventricular preload • Reduction in edema and cardiac size causes an increase in cardiac efficiency	• Treatment of mild to moderate CHF • Often used in combination with dietary sodium restriction	• Hypercalcemia • Hyperglycemia • Hyperlipidemia • Hypermagnesemia • Hyperuricemia • Hypokalemia • Hyponatremia • Metabolic alkalosis • Muscle weakness • Pancreatitis • Vasodilation
Loop Diuretic				
Furosemide (Lasix)	• **A:** IV, IM, and PO • **M:** Metabolized to a small degree in the liver • **E:** Metabolite and parent drug excreted in urine		• Acute and chronic treatment of severe CHF (when thiazide diuretics are no longer effective)	• Hyperglycemia • Hyperuricemia • Hypocalcemia or hypercalcemia • Hypokalemia • Hyponatremia • Hypomagnesemia

Continued

6. Medications Affecting Cardiac and Renal Function

CHF THERAPY: DIURETICS AND ACE INHIBITORS (Continued)

Drug	Pharmacokinetics	Mechanism of Action	Clinical Uses	Side Effects
Potassium-Sparing Diuretic				
Spironolactone (Aldactone)	• **A:** PO • **M:** Metabolized to active metabolites • **E:** Majority of metabolites excreted in urine; remaining in feces		• Chronic treatment of CHF • Increased aldosterone states	• Hyperkalemia (especially with ACE inhibitors, angiotensin receptor blockers, β-blockers and NSAIDs) • CNS depression causing drowsiness • Metabolic acidosis • Gynecomastia
ACE Inhibitors				
Captopril (Capoten)	• **A:** PO • **M:** Prodrugs converted by liver to active metabolites • **E:** In urine	• Reduce peripheral resistance and, thus, afterload • Reduce aldosterone release, which decreases water and salt retention, thus, decreasing preload • Reduction in angiotensin II can lead to a decrease in sympathetic activity • Reduce long-term remodeling of the heart	• Long-term treatment of CHF • Also used in the treatment of hypertension	☞ CAPTOPRIL **C**ough **A**ngioedema **P**roteinuria **T**aste changes Hyp**O**tension **P**regnancy problems (teratogenic) **R**ash **I**ncrease renin **L**ower angiotensin II
Enalapril (Vasotec)	• **A:** IV and PO • **E:** Unchanged in urine			

IV. Medications that Affect Angiotensin Action

DRUGS THAT INTERFERE WITH THE ACTION OF ANGIOTENSIN

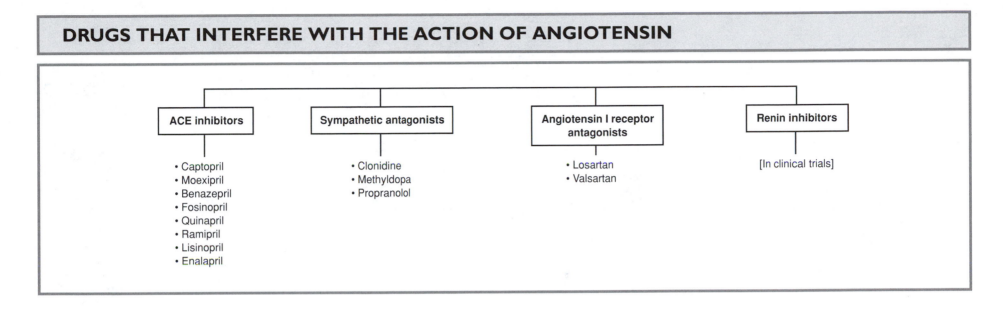

ACE inhibitors	Sympathetic antagonists	Angiotensin I receptor antagonists	Renin inhibitors
• Captopril	• Clonidine	• Losartan	[In clinical trials]
• Moexipril	• Methyldopa	• Valsartan	
• Benazepril	• Propranolol		
• Fosinopril			
• Quinapril			
• Ramipril			
• Lisinopril			
• Enalapril			

DRUGS THAT AFFECT ANGIOTENSIN ACTION

Drug	Pharmacokinetics	Mechanism of Action	Clinical Uses	Drawbacks and Side Effects
ACE Inhibitors				
Captopril (Capoten)	• **A:** PO • **M:** Prodrugs converted by liver to active metabolites • **E:** In urine (except fosinopril and moexipril, which are also excreted in feces)	• Inhibit the formation of the potent vasoconstrictor angiotensin II from angiotensin I by the inhibition ACE • Primarily decrease peripheral vascular resistance • Reduce the breakdown of bradykinin	• Hypertension • CHF • Diabetic neuropathy • Post MI (unlike direct vasoconstrictors, these drugs do not induce reflex sympathetic activation and, thus, can be used in patients with ischemic heart disease) • Increase in bradykinin can contribute to vasodilation	• Dry cough and skin rash (due to increase in bradykinin levels caused by the inhibition of ACE) • Hyperkalemia (especially seen in patients also on potassium-sparing diuretics) • Acute renal failure (due to reduced glomerular filtration rate) • Teratogenic (do not administer to pregnant women in their second or third trimesters) • Neutropenia • Hypotension
Moexipril (Univasc)				
Benazepril (Lotensin)				
Fosinopril (Monopril)				
Quinapril (Accupril)				
Ramipril (Altace)	• **A:** PO • **M:** Hepatic metabolism to active and inactive metabolites • **E:** Parent drug and metabolites excreted in urine and feces			
Lisinopril (Prinivil, Zestril)	• **A:** PO • **E:** Unchanged in urine			
Enalapril (Vasotec)	• **A:** IV and PO • **E:** Unchanged in urine			

Sympathetic Antagonists

Clonidine (Catapres)	• **A:** PO and transdermal • **M:** 50% hepatic metabolism • **E:** Majority excreted unchanged in urine	• Inhibit renin release by inhibiting the sympathetic nervous system • Renin release is the rate-limiting step in the renin-angiotensin system	• Hypertension • CHF	• Many adverse effects associated with the inhibition of the sympathetic nervous system due to nonselective nature of these medications • Bronchoconstriction • Hypotension • Bradycardia • Sexual dysfunction
Methyldopa (Aldomet)	• **A:** PO and IV • **M:** Hepatic metabolism • **E:** Parent drug and metabolites excreted in urine			
Propranolol (Inderal)	• **A:** PO and IV; well absorbed • **M:** Hepatic metabolism • **E:** Metabolites excreted in urine			

Angiotensin Receptor Blockers

Losartan (Cozaar)	• **A:** PO • **M:** Extensive first-pass hepatic metabolism by P450 system • **E:** Parent drug and metabolite excreted in urine and feces	• Block the angiotensin I receptor so that angiotensin II cannot bind and have any effect	• Hypertension • CHF	• Smaller incidence of side effects than ACE inhibitors • No bradykinin increase (no cough or rash)
Valsartan (Diovan)	• **A:** PO • **M:** Minor hepatic metabolism by P450 system • **E:** Parent drug and metabolite excreted in urine and feces			

Renin Inhibitors

N/A	• N/A	• Block the action of renin on angiotensinogen, thus blocking the formation of angiotensin I • Theoretically will inhibit step 1	• Intended for the treatment of hypertension and CHF	• Very low bioavailability • Still in clinical trial stage

THE FUNCTIONS OF ANGIOTENSIN

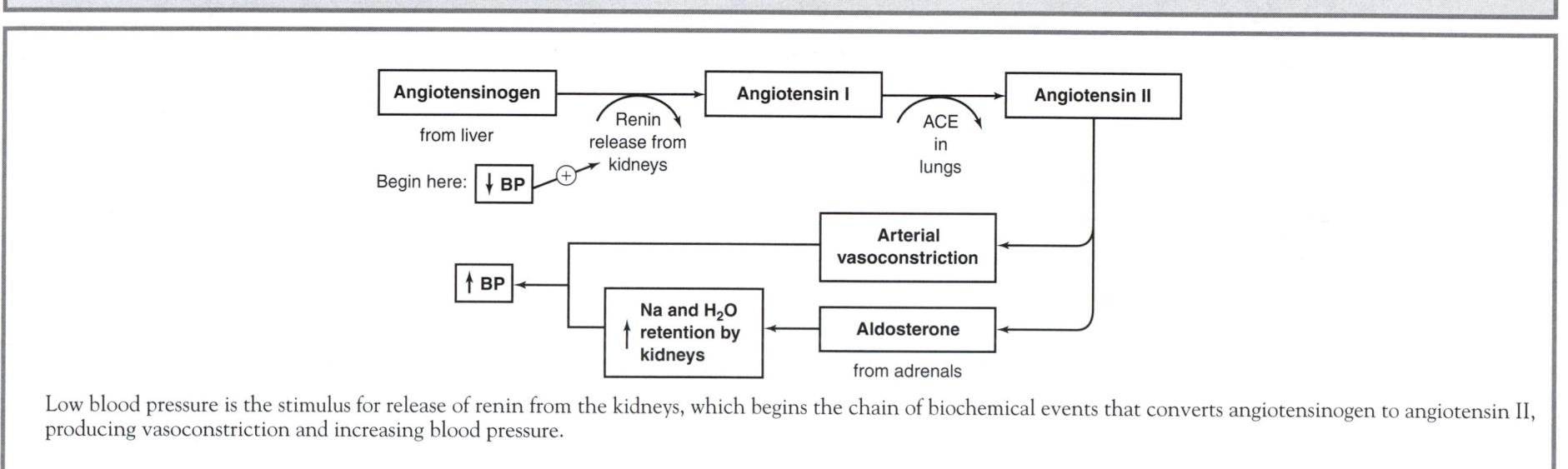

Low blood pressure is the stimulus for release of renin from the kidneys, which begins the chain of biochemical events that converts angiotensinogen to angiotensin II, producing vasoconstriction and increasing blood pressure.

V. Antihypertensive Drugs

CLASSIFICATION OF ANTIHYPERTENSIVE DRUGS

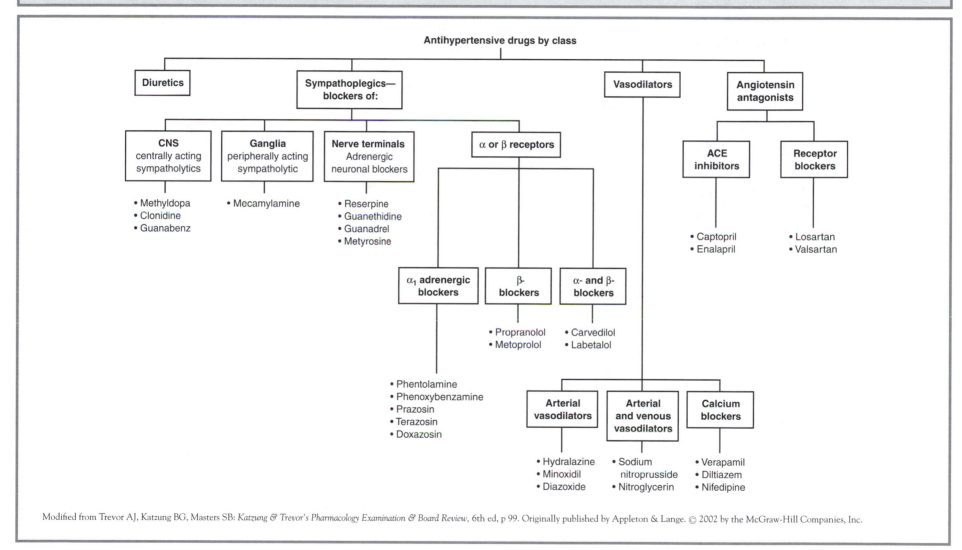

Modified from Trevor AJ, Katzung BG, Masters SB: *Katzung & Trevor's Pharmacology Examination & Board Review*, 6th ed, p 99. Originally published by Appleton & Lange. © 2002 by the McGraw-Hill Companies, Inc.

ANTIHYPERTENSIVES: SYMPATHOLYTICS

Drug	Pharmacokinetics	Mechanism of Action	Clinical Uses	Side Effects
Centrally Acting Sympatholytic				
Methyldopa (Aldomet)	• **A:** PO and IV • **M:** Hepatic metabolism • **E:** Parent drug and metabolites excreted in urine	• Believed to work in the relay area of the solitary nucleus • Act as α_2-receptor agonists to reduce sympathetic tone to peripheral structures (decrease peripheral resistance, HR, and plasma renin activity)	• Hypertension • CHF	• Plasma volume is increased (body's attempt to reestablish homeostasis) leading to mild edema • Sedation, dizziness, and headache (diminish as tolerance develops) • Mild bradycardia • Flu-like symptoms with fever • Lupus-like syndrome • Positive Coombs' test with no increase in hemolytic anemia
Clonidine (Catapres)	• **A:** PO and transdermal patch (good for noncompliant patients; provides steady-state blood levels, also fewer side effects) • **M:** 50% hepatic metabolism • **E:** Majority excreted unchanged in urine		• Hypertension • As effective as methyldopa but requires smaller doses • CHF	• High dose will cause interaction with α_1-receptors leading to vasoconstriction and increased BP • Drowsiness, dizziness, and headache (subside with tolerance) • Plasma volume is increased (body's attempt to reestablish homeostasis) leading to mild edema • Mild bradycardia • Xerostomia • Constipation • Patch can cause itching, irritation, and redness

Guanabenz (Wytensin)	• **A:** PO • **M:** Site of metabolism unknown • **E:** Metabolites excreted in urine		• Hypertension • Often combined with thiazide diuretics	• Confusion/mental depression • Antimuscarinic side effects • Headache • Nausea

Peripherally Acting Sympatholytic

Mecamylamine (Inversine)	• **A:** PO • **E:** Unchanged in urine	• Nondepolarizing ganglionic blocker • Competitive inhibitor of Ach at nicotinic receptors on postganglionic autonomic neurons • Blocks sympathetic ganglia causing vasodilation and decreased HR	• Hypertension (numerous side effects preclude its common use)	• CNS side effects (convulsions, mental changes, tremors, confusion) • Hypotension

ANTIHYPERTENSIVES: ADRENERGIC BLOCKERS

Drug	Pharmacokinetics	Mechanism of Action	Clinical Uses	Side Effects
Adrenergic Neuronal Blockers				
Reserpine (Serpasil)	• **A:** PO • **M:** Hepatic metabolism • **E:** Parent drug and metabolites excreted in urine and feces	• Blocks reuptake of NE and DA into vesicle within the neuron by inhibiting Mg ATPase • Depletion of NT leads to decreased activity in blood vessels and heart	• Mild hypertension • Used only rarely (due to CNS side effects) in small doses with other drugs like diuretics and β-blockers	• Severe depression • Suicide • Sedation • Bradycardia
Guanethidine (Ismelin) Guanadrel (Hylorel)	• **A:** PO • **M:** Hepatic metabolism • **E:** Parent drug and metabolites excreted in urine	• Replaces NE bound to ATP in vesicles • Results in decreased NE released with nerve stimulation • Leads to reduced arteriolar vasoconstriction	• Moderate to severe hypertension	• Angina • Edema (peripheral and pulmonary) • Fatigue • Severe diarrhea
Metyrosine (Demser)	• **A:** PO • **M:** Majority excreted unchanged in urine	• Competitive inhibitor of tyrosine hydroxylase • Reduces synthesis of NE and EPI causing decreased BP	• Prophylaxis and treatment of hypertension associated with pheochromocytomectomy • Chronic treatment for malignant pheochromocytoma	• Severe diarrhea • EPS (see section on antipsychotics in Chapter 4 for more information) • Allergic reactions
Nonselective α-Adrenergic Blockers				
Phentolamine (Regitine, Rogitine)	• **A:** IM, IV • **M:** Not well defined; reversible • **E:** Not well defined; some excreted unchanged in urine	• α-Adrenergic blockade leads to decreased systemic vascular resistance • Results in decreased BP	• Diagnosis of pheochromocytoma • Prophylaxis and treatment of hypertension associated with pheochromocytomectomy	• Reflex tachycardia • Orthostatic hypotension • GI disturbances (nausea, diarrhea) • Weakness

Phenoxy-benzamine (Dibenzyline)	• **A:** PO • **M:** Hepatic metabolism; irreversible • **E:** Metabolites excreted in urine and feces		• As above • BPH	

Selective α-Adrenergic Blockers

Prazosin (Minipress)	• **A:** PO • **M:** Hepatic metabolism to active metabolites • **E:** Parent drug and metabolites excreted in bile and feces		• Hypertension • BPH • Cause less reflex tachycardia than nonselective α-adrenergic blockers	• First dose orthostatic hypotension (can lead to syncope) requires careful dosing (usually before bed) • Dizziness • Drowsiness (will subside) • Headache • Peripheral edema • Palpitations
Terazosin (Hytrin)	• **A:** PO • **M:** Hepatic metabolism to active metabolites • **E:** Parent drug and metabolites excreted in urine and feces			
Doxazosin (Cardura)	• **A:** PO • **M:** Hepatic metabolism • **E:** Parent drug and metabolites excreted in bile and feces			

ANTIHYPERTENSIVES: β-BLOCKERS

Drug	Pharmacokinetics	Mechanism of Action	Clinical Uses	Side Effects
Propranolol (Inderal)	• **A:** PO and IV; well absorbed • **M:** Hepatic metabolism • **E:** Metabolites excreted in urine	• Nonselective β-blocker • Blocks β_1-receptors in the heart, increasing sympathetic activity and decreasing BP • β_1-Blockade of the juxtaglomerular apparatus leads to decreased renin release (less angiotensin formation)	• Hypertension • Other uses include angina, cardiac arrhythmias, migraine, acute MI, essential tremor	• Contraindicated in patients with asthma, COPD, diabetes mellitus, or peripheral vascular disease • Bronchoconstriction • Hypotension • Bradycardia • Sexual dysfunction
Metoprolol (Lopressor, Toprol)		• Selective β_1-blocker • Same as above	• Hypertension • Other uses include angina, CHF, acute MI • Less side effects than nonselective β-blocker	
Labetalol (Normodyne, Trandate)	• **A:** PO and IV • **M:** Hepatic metabolism • **E:** Parent drug and metabolites excreted in urine and feces	• Nonselective β-blocker (predominant activity) with selective α_1-blocker activity • Decreases HR, decreases plasma renin activity, and increases plasma volume (β-blockade) • Decreases peripheral vascular resistance (α blockade) • α-Blocker activity counteracts vasoconstriction that leads to cold toes and fingers that is associated with β-blockers	• Hypertension	• Postural hypotension • Dizziness • Nausea • Fatigue
Carvedilol (Coreg)	• **A:** PO • **M:** Extensive first-pass hepatic metabolism; metabolized by P450 enzymes • **E:** Metabolites excreted in feces	• β- and α-Blocker • Similar actions as labetalol	• Hypertension • CHF	• Bradycardia • Dizziness • Hypotension

ANTIHYPERTENSIVES: VASODILATORS

Drug	Pharmacokinetics	Mechanism of Action	Clinical Uses	Side Effects
Arterial Vasodilators				
Hydralazine (Apresoline)	• **A:** PO, IM, and IV • **M:** Extensive first-pass hepatic metabolism; hepatic acetylation (remember that certain patient populations have varying rates of acetylation) • **E:** Metabolites excreted in urine	• Arterial smooth muscle relaxation and vasodilation (probably through action on cAMP and Ca^{2+})	• Hypertension • CHF	• Toxicity in slow acetylators • Tachycardia • Headache • Dizziness • Nausea • Sweating • Flushing • Nasal congestion • Lupus-like syndrome
Minoxidil (Loniten)	• **A:** PO and topical • **M:** Hepatic metabolism • **E:** Metabolites excreted in urine	• Inhibits PDE leading to increased levels of cAMP, which through Ca^{2+} modulation leads to arterial smooth muscle relaxation and vasodilation	• Hypertension • Alopecia	• Tachycardia • Massive fluid retention • Hypertrichosis (hair growth) • ECG changes • Pericarditis
Diazoxide (Proglycem, Hyperstat)	• **A:** PO or IV • **M:** Partial hepatic metabolism • **E:** Parent drug and metabolites excreted in urine	• Decreases peripheral vascular resistance via direct vasodilatory effect on smooth muscle in peripheral arterioles	• Acute hypertensive emergencies • Hypoglycemia (secondary to hyperinsulinemia via inhibition of insulin release)	• Reflex tachycardia

Continued

ANTIHYPERTENSIVES: VASODILATORS (Continued)

Drug	Pharmacokinetics	Mechanism of Action	Clinical Uses	Side Effects
Arterial and Venous Vasodilator				
Sodium nitroprusside (Nitropress, Nipride)	• **A:** IV • **M:** Local metabolism by tissues and erythrocytes • **E:** Metabolites excreted in urine, feces, and exhaled air	• Dilates arteries and veins	• Acute hypertensive emergencies • CHF	• Byproduct of metabolism is cyanide, which is metabolized by the liver by rhodanase to thiocyanate (water soluble and excreted in urine) • Cyanide poisoning in patients with poor diets (alcoholics) where it leads to decreased sulfur availability or when administered in high doses for long period of time • Drug is broken down by UV light so IV bag must be wrapped in foil
Nitroglycerin (Nitro-Bid, Nitro-Dur, Nitrogard)	• **A:** Sublingual, PO, IV, ointment, or patches • **M:** Hepatic metabolism to active metabolites	• Converted to nitric oxide intracellularly, which activates guanylate cyclase, leading to the following cascade of events: – leading to an increase in cGMP – causing dephosphorylation of myosin light chain – leading to relaxation of vascular smooth muscle resulting in vasodilation	• Advantages over sodium nitroprusside: not light sensitive, inexpensive, readily available, no cyanide toxicity	• Headache • Repeated administration leads to a loss of effectiveness • Large degree of cross tolerance between organic nitrates • Systemic compensation (salt and water retention) may also be involved in loss of effectiveness

Drug	Pharmacokinetics	Mechanism of Action	Clinical Uses	Side Effects
Calcium Channel Blockers				
Verapamil (Calan, Isoptin)	• **A:** PO and IV • **M:** Extensive first-pass hepatic metabolism; metabolized by P450 enzymes to active metabolite • **E:** In urine and feces	• Block voltage sensitive calcium channels located primarily in the cardiac muscle and in vascular smooth muscle causing decrease in IC Ca^{2+} • Also block cyclic nucleotide PDE, which increases cGMP and decreases Ca^{2+} influx • Results in dilation of peripheral arterioles and venules	• Hypertension • Angina • Antiarrhythmic	• Peripheral edema • Hypotension • Palpitations due to reflex tachycardia • Dizziness and headaches • Constipation • Nausea • Abdominal cramps
Diltiazem (Cardizem)	• **A:** PO and IV • **M:** Extensive first-pass hepatic metabolism; metabolized by P450 enzymes to less active metabolites • **E:** In urine and feces			
Nifedipine (Adalat, Procardia)	• **A:** PO • **M:** Extensive first-pass hepatic metabolism; metabolized by P450 enzymes to inactive metabolites • **E:** In urine and feces		• Hypertension • Angina	

Continued

ANTIHYPERTENSIVES: CALCIUM CHANNEL BLOCKERS AND ANGIOTENSIN ANTAGONISTS (Continued)

Drug	Pharmacokinetics	Mechanism of Action	Clinical Uses	Side Effects
ACE Inhibitors				
Captopril (Capoten)	• **A:** PO • **M:** Prodrugs converted by liver to active metabolites • **E:** In urine	• Decrease BP by inhibiting the enzyme responsible for production of angiotensin II, a potent vasoconstrictor • Also prevents breakdown of bradykinin, a vasodilator	• Hypertension • CHF	• Bradykinin increase leading to cough and skin rash • Teratogenesis • Hyperkalemia • Neutropenia • Hypotension • Acute renal failure
Enalapril (Vasotec)	• **A:** IV and PO • **E:** Unchanged in urine			
Angiotensin Receptor Blockers				
Losartan (Cozaar)	• **A:** PO • **M:** Hepatic metabolism by P450 system • **E:** Parent drug and metabolite excreted in urine and feces	• Angiotensin I receptor blockade prevents the vasoconstriction caused by angiotensin I	• Hypertension • CHF	• Smaller incidence of side effects than ACE inhibitor • No bradykinin increase (no cough or rash)
Valsartan (Diovan)				

VI. Diuretics

CLASSIFICATION OF DIURETICS

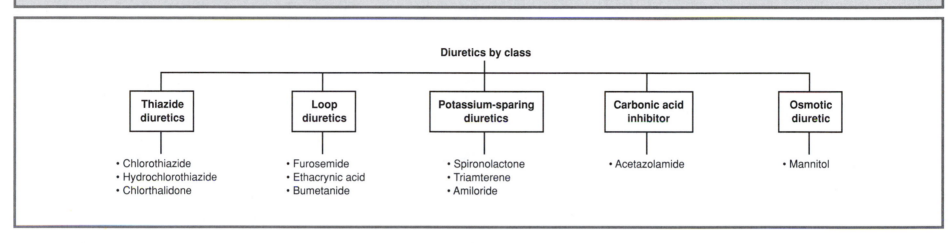

Diuretics by class

Thiazide diuretics	Loop diuretics	Potassium-sparing diuretics	Carbonic acid inhibitor	Osmotic diuretic
• Chlorothiazide • Hydrochlorothiazide • Chlorthalidone	• Furosemide • Ethacrynic acid • Bumetanide	• Spironolactone • Triamterene • Amiloride	• Acetazolamide	• Mannitol

THIAZIDE, LOOP, AND POTASSIUM-SPARING DIURETICS

Drug	Pharmacokinetics	Mechanism of Action	Clinical Uses and General Information	Side Effects
Thiazide Diuretics				
Chlorothiazide (Diuril)	• **A:** PO and IV • **DOA:** 6–12 hours • **E:** Unchanged in urine • **Urine chemistry (opposite of blood chemistry):** Increased Na^+, Cl^-, K^+, water, and Mg^{2+}; decreased Ca^{2+} and pH	• Increase urinary and salt output by inhibiting Na^+ and Cl^- reabsorption in the distal tubule	• Hypertension • CHF • Nephrolithiasis due to hypercalciuria • Diabetes insipidus	• Hypercalcemia • Hyperglycemia • Hyperlipidemia • Hypomagnesemia • Hyperuricemia (increased risk for gout) • Hypokalemia • Hyponatremia • Metabolic alkalosis • Muscle weakness (due to loss of salt) • Pancreatitis (decreased insulin release) • Vasodilation
Hydrochlorothiazide (HydroDIURIL, HCTZ)	• **A:** PO • **DOA:** 6–12 hours • **E:** Unchanged in urine			
Chlorthalidone (Hygroton)	• **A:** PO • **DOA:** 48–72 hours • **E:** Unchanged in urine			

Loop Diuretics

Furosemide (Lasix)	• **A:** IV, IM, and PO • **DOA:** 6–8 hours • **M:** Metabolized to a small degree in the liver • **E:** Metabolite and parent drug excreted in urine • **Urine chemistry:** Increased Na^+, Cl^-, K^+, water, Ca^{2+}, Mg^{2+}; decreased HCO_3^- and pH	• Block reabsorption of Na^+ and Cl^- in the cortex and medullary regions of the ascending loop of Henle	• Hyperkalemia • Acute hypertension states • Drugs of choice for edematous situations • Acute renal failure • Hypercalcemia • 10 times more efficacious than thiazide diuretics	• Hyperglycemia: similar effect on pancreas as thiazides • Hyperuricemia • Hypocalcemia or hypercalcemia • Hypokalemia • Hypokalemic metabolic acidosis • Hyponatremia • Hypomagnesemia • Ototoxicity (reversible tinnitus) • Interstitial nephritis
Ethacrynic Acid (Edecrin)	• **A:** IV and PO • **M:** Hepatic metabolism • **E:** Parent drug and metabolite excreted in urine and feces			
Bumetanide (Bumex)	• **A:** IV, IM, and PO • **M:** Partial hepatic metabolism • **E:** Parent drug and metabolite excreted in urine and feces			

Continued

THIAZIDE, LOOP, AND POTASSIUM-SPARING DIURETICS (Continued)

Drug	Pharmacokinetics	Mechanism of Action	Clinical Uses and General Information	Side Effects
Potassium-Sparing Diuretics				
Spironolactone (Aldactone)	• **A:** PO • **M:** Metabolized to active metabolites • **E:** Majority of metabolites excreted in urine; remaining excreted in feces • **Urine chemistry:** K^+ is lower than Na^+	• Blocks the effects of aldosterone in the collecting duct leading to Na^+ loss and K^+ retention	• Increased aldosterone states (Conn's syndrome, ectopic ACTH production, or secondary hyperaldosteronism due to CHF, nephrotic syndrome, or hepatic cirrhosis) • Often combined with thiazides to treat hypertension and prevent hypokalemia	• Hyperkalemia (especially with ACE inhibitors, angiotensin receptor blockers, β-blockers, and NSAIDs) • CNS depression causing drowsiness • Metabolic acidosis • Gynecomastia with spironolactone • Nephrolithasis with triamterene
Triamterene (Dyrenium)	• **A:** PO • **M:** Hepatic metabolism • **E:** Parent drug and metabolites excreted in urine	• Retain K^+ and excrete Na^+ in the collecting duct but does not work on aldosterone		
Amiloride (Midamor)	• **A:** PO • **E:** Unchanged in urine and feces			

CARBONIC ACID INHIBITOR AND OSMOTIC DIURETICS

Drug	Pharmacokinetics	Mechanism of Action	Clinical Uses	Side Effects
Carbonic Acid Inhibitor (CAI) Diuretic				
Acetazolamide (Diamox)	• **A:** PO and IV • **E:** Unchanged in urine • **Urine chemistry:** Increased Na^+, HCO_3^-, water, pH, K^+; decreased Cl^-	• Prevents the reabsorption of bicarbonate at the proximal convoluted tubule • Na^+ increases in the urine because H^+ is no longer being excreted to combine with HCO_3^-	• Glaucoma (carbonic anhydrase is important in the production of aqueous humor) • Metabolic alkalosis • Altitude sickness	• Paresthesias • Tinnitis • GI upset • Hyperchloremic metabolic acidosis • Neuropathy • Ammonia toxicity • Sulfa drug allergy
Osmotic Diuretic				
Mannitol (Osmitrol)	• **A:** IV • **M:** Metabolized to a minor degree in the liver to glycogen • **E:** Most is excreted unchanged in urine	• Raises solutes in the blood causing hypertonic blood, which draws fluid out of the tissues • Increased plasma volume will deliver more volume to the kidney leading to increased GFR, which leads to increased urinary output	• Reduction of intraocular or intracranial pressure (CNS trauma with swelling and edema) • Maintain urinary output for renal protection (ie, rhabdomyolysis or hemolysis) • Acute altitude sickness ☞ Good for head swelling, bad for heart swelling	• Transiently causes increased intravascular pressure, which can exacerbate CHF or hypertension • Dehydration • Hypernatremia

SERUM ELECTROLYTE EFFECTS OF DIURETICS

In general, the opposite findings of serum electrolytes are seen in urine.

Type of Diuretic	Ca	Mg	Na	K	Uric Acid	Blood Sugar	Lipids	Metabolic Disturbance
Thiazide	↑	↓	↓	↓	↑	↑	↑	Hypokalemic metabolic alkalosis
Loop	↓	↓	↓	↓	↑	↑	—	
Potassium-sparing	—	↑	↓	↑	↑	—	—	Hyperchloremic metabolic acidosis
CAI	—	—	—	↓	↑	↑	—	

VII. Antihyperlipidemic Drugs

CLASSIFICATION OF ANTIHYPERLIPIDEMIC DRUGS

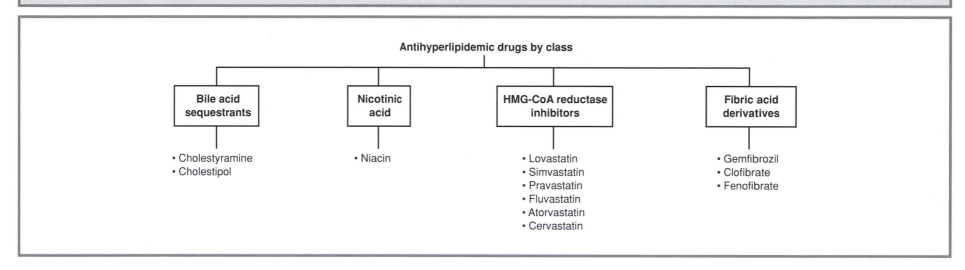

Antihyperlipidemic drugs by class

Bile acid sequestrants	Nicotinic acid	HMG-CoA reductase inhibitors	Fibric acid derivatives
• Cholestyramine • Cholestipol	• Niacin	• Lovastatin • Simvastatin • Pravastatin • Fluvastatin • Atorvastatin • Cervastatin	• Gemfibrozil • Clofibrate • Fenofibrate

ANTIHYPERLIPIDEMICS: BILE ACID SEQUESTRANTS AND NICOTINIC ACID

Drug	Pharmacokinetics	Mechanism of Action	Clinical Uses	Side Effects
Bile Acid Sequestrants				
Cholestyramine (Questran) Cholestipol (Cholestid)	• **A:** PO • **E:** Drug/bile acid complex is excreted in feces	• Anion exchange resin that binds bile acids in the intestine and prevents reabsorption • Reduction in bile acid reabsorption results in an increase in production of bile acids from cholesterol in the liver • This increased demand for cholesterol by the liver increases the expression of LDL receptors by the liver • LDL is cleared from the plasma more quickly due to the increased population of receptors	• Greatest effect is seen at lowest doses of the drug • Decreases LDL 10–30% • Increases HDL 2–4% • Increases VLDL-TG levels 5–30% • No effect on Lp(a)	• Abdominal pain • Bloating • Constipation • Pancreatitis • Interference with absorption of fat soluble vitamins (A, E, D, K) • Binds to HMG-CoA reductase inhibitors
Nicotinic Acid				
Niacin (Niaspan, Nicolar)	• **A:** PO; rapidly absorbed • **M:** Extensive first-pass hepatic metabolism • **E:** Metabolites and parent drug excreted in urine	• Decreases the production of VLDL • Increases circulating levels of HDL • Decreases Lp(a)	• Decreases LDL 10–25% • Decreases VLDL-TG 50% • Increases HDL 30–40%	• Acanthosis nigricans • Aggravation of asthma • Atrial arrhythmias • Cutaneous flushing • Gastritis/ulcer disease • Glucose intolerance • Hepatitis • Hyperuricemia • Increased risk of hepatotoxicity at dose required for sustained release formula: adjust dose when switching from sustained release form to normal oral form

ANTIHYPERLIPIDEMICS: HMG-CoA REDUCTASE INHIBITORS

Drug	Pharmacokinetics	Mechanism of Action	Clinical Uses	Side Effects
Lovastatin (Mevacor) Simvastatin (Zocor) Pravastatin (Pravachol) Fluvastatin (Lescol) Atorvastatin (Lipitor)	• **A:** PO; well absorbed • **M:** Extensive first-pass hepatic metabolism • **E:** Parent drug and metabolites excreted in urine and feces	• Inhibits HMG-CoA reductase, the enzyme required for cholesterol synthesis • Increased production of LDL receptors in the liver • Increased uptake of LDL from the plasma • Decreases VLDL secretion	• Decreases LDL 20–50% • Decreases TG 10–20% • Increases HDL 5–10% • No effect on Lp(a)	• Elevated liver transaminases (3 times normal) • Headaches • Myopathy (uncommon and dose dependent) • Cataracts (unproven)

ANTIHYPERLIPIDEMIC: FIBRIC ACID DERIVATIVES

Drug	Pharmacokinetics	Mechanism of Action	Clinical Uses	Side Effects
Gemfibrozil (Lopid)	• **A:** PO; well absorbed • **M:** Hepatic metabolism • **E:** Parent drug and metabolites excreted in urine	• Unknown but may increase the activity of LP lipase, thereby increasing the catabolism of VLDL • May inhibit lipolysis of stored fat and decrease hepatic extraction of free fatty acids • Stimulate the production of Apo A-1, the major protein component of HDL	• Decreases VLDL-TG 40–55% • Decreases LDL < 10% • Increases HDL 20% • May decrease platelet reactivity and aggregability and concentration of fibrinogen	• Alopecia • Decreased libido • Drowsiness • GI distress • Lithogenicity of bile • Myositis • Neutropenia • Ventricular arrhythmias (clofibrate) • Weight gain • LTU can lead to increased gallbladder toxicity, increased appendectomies, hepatotoxicity (fenofibrate), and potential risk for human carcinogenesis
Clofibrate (Atromid)	• **A:** PO; well absorbed • **M:** Metabolized by serum enzymes then conjugated in liver • **E:** Metabolites excreted in urine			
Fenofibrate (Tricor)	• **A:** PO • **M:** Hepatic metabolism to active metabolite • **E:** Metabolites excreted in urine			

SUMMARY OF ANTIHYPERLIPIDEMIC DRUG EFFECTS

(Shading indicates presence of effect.)

Drug Class	Decrease Cholesterol Synthesis	Increase Peripheral Apo B and E Receptors	Bind Bile Acids in Gut, Increase Enterohepatic Circulation	Enhance VLDL/LDL Breakdown	Lower VLDL Synthesis	Increase HDL Synthesis	Lower Lp(a)
Bile acid sequestrants		■	■				
Nicotinic acid					■		■
HMG-CoA reductase inhibitors	■	■					
Fibric acid derivatives		■		■		■	

EFFECTS OF ANTIHYPERLIPIDEMICS ON LIPOPROTEINS

Drug Class	LDL	HDL	VLDL-TG
Bile acid sequestrants	↓	↑	↑
Nicotinic acid	↓	↑	↓
HMG-CoA reductase inhibitors	↓	↑	↓ (TG)
Fibric acid derivatives	↓	↑	↓

VIII. Managing Coagulopathy

DRUGS USED IN CLOTTING DISORDERS

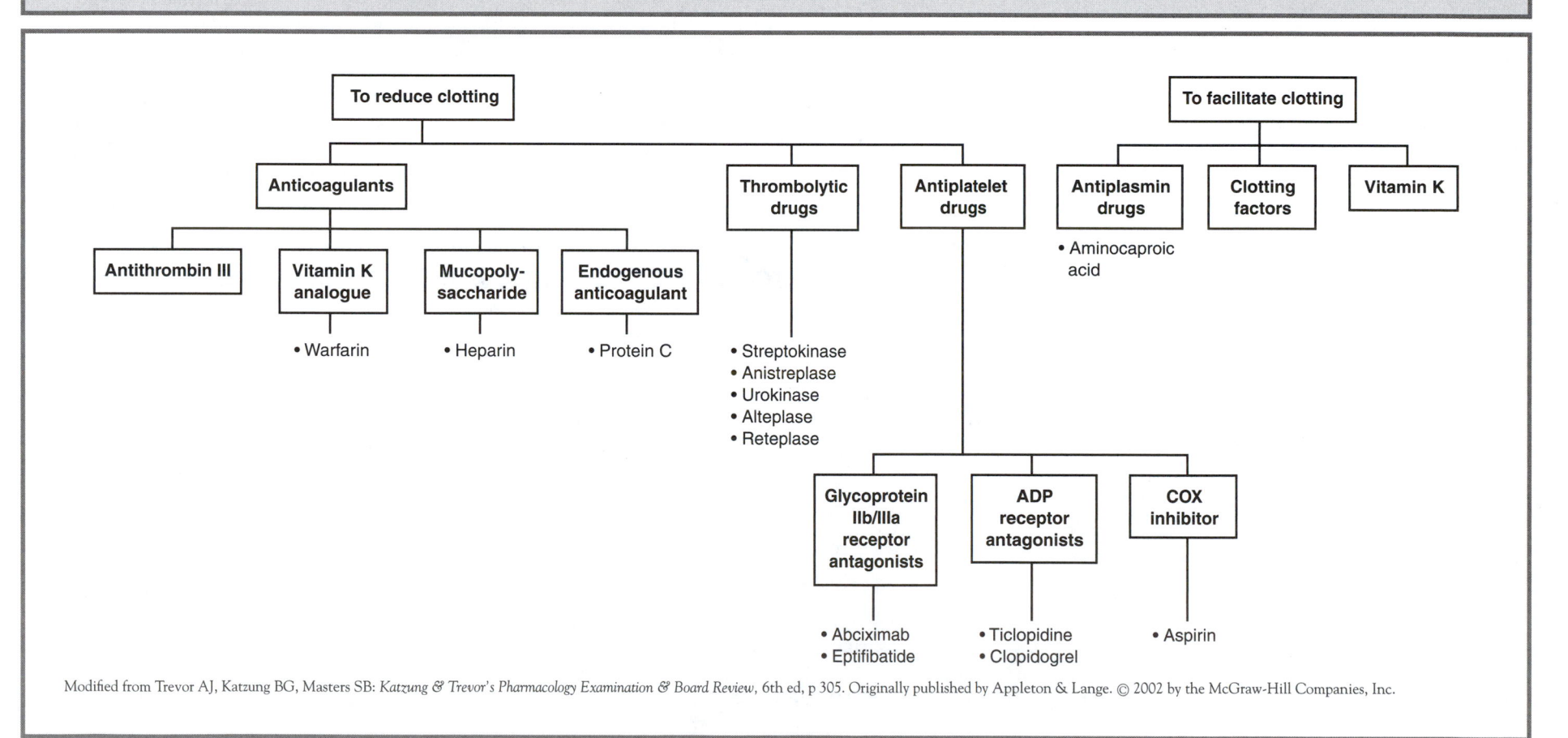

Modified from Trevor AJ, Katzung BG, Masters SB: *Katzung & Trevor's Pharmacology Examination & Board Review*, 6th ed, p 305. Originally published by Appleton & Lange. © 2002 by the McGraw-Hill Companies, Inc.

DRUGS USED TO REDUCE CLOTTING: ANTICOAGULANTS, THROMBOLYTICS, AND ANTIPLATELETS

Drug	Pharmacokinetics	Mechanism of Action	Clinical Uses	Side Effects
Anticoagulants				
Heparin (Hepalean)	• **A:** IV or SC • **D:** Does not cross the placenta • **M:** Unknown (may be partially metabolized by liver and reticuloendothelial system) • **E:** Small amount excreted unchanged in urine	• Binds to and activates endogenous antithrombin III, which acts to inhibit clotting factors VII, IX, X, and II	• Acute anticoagulation • Reversed with protamine sulfate • Effectiveness monitored by PTT level • New low-molecular-weight (LMW) heparins have longer DOA allowing for once a day dosing	• Excessive bleeding • Thrombocytopenia • Alopecia • LTU can lead to osteoporosis and spontaneous fracture
Warfarin (Coumadin)	• **A:** PO • **B:** 99% protein bound • **D:** Widely distributed; crosses placenta • **M:** Hepatic P450 metabolism	• Blocks reduction of vitamin K necessary for carboxylation of coagulation factors • Inhibits synthesis of VII, IX, X, and II	• Chronic anticoagulation • Reversed with vitamin K and/or factor IX • Effectiveness monitored by prothrombin time level	• Contraindicated in pregnant women • Excessive bleeding • Causes cutaneous necrosis • Rarely causes frank infarction of breast, fatty tissues, bowel, or extremities (purple toe syndrome)
Protein C	• N/A	• Activated by thrombomodulin from endothelial cells • Decreases factors V, VIII, and XI	• Endogeneous self-modulating mechanism	• None

Continued

DRUGS USED TO REDUCE CLOTTING: ANTICOAGULANTS, THROMBOLYTICS, AND ANTIPLATELETS (Continued)

Drug	Pharmacokinetics	Mechanism of Action	Clinical Uses	Side Effects
Thrombolytics				
Streptokinase (Kabikinase, Streptase)	• **A:** IV • **E:** Cleared from blood by antibodies and reticuloendothelial system	• Protein from *Streptococcus* that converts plasminogen to plasmin • Plasmin then functions to break up the clot by dissolving fibrin	• IV for multiple pulmonary emboli or central deep venous thrombosis • Management of acute MIs • t-PA is also utilized for patients with acute stroke symptoms (shown to decrease neurologic disability at 1-year post CVA)	• Excessive bleeding • Cerebral hemorrhage • Fever, allergic reactions, and therapeutic resistance in patients with streptococcal antibodies
Anistreplase (Eminase)	• **A:** IV • **M:** Breaks down into components following administration	• Human plasminogen and bacterial streptokinase that has been acylated to protect the enzyme's active site		• Excessive bleeding • Cerebral hemorrhage
Urokinase (Abbokinase)	• **A:** IV • **M:** Rapidly cleared from blood • **E:** Small amount excreted in urine and feces	• Human enzyme produced by the kidney that converts plasminogen to plasmin • Plasmin then functions to break up the clot by dissolving fibrin		
Alteplase (Activase)	• **A:** IV • **M:** Principally cleared by liver • **E:** In urine	• Unmodified human tissue plasminogen activator (t-PA) • Converts fibrin-bound plasminogen to plasmin (clot selective)		
Reteplase (Retavase)	• **A:** IV • **E:** Cleared by kidneys and liver	• Human t-PA from which several amino acids have been deleted • Converts fibrin-bound plasminogen to plasmin (clot selective)		

Antiplatelets

Aspirin (Ecotrin, Bayer)	• **A:** PO • **M:** Extensive first-pass hepatic metabolism • **E:** Metabolites excreted in urine	• Prevents activation of thromboxane A_2 (a potent stimulator of platelet aggregation) by irreversibly binding to COX	• Prevention of MIs	• Excessive bleeding • GI bleeding • PUD
Abciximab (Reopro)	• **A:** IV • **E:** Rapidly cleared from blood (likely secondary to rapid receptor binding)	• Human monoclonal antibody directed against the glycoprotein IIb/IIIa complex	• Prevention of restenosis after angioplasty • Acute coronary syndrome (unstable angina or non–Q wave acute MI)	• Excessive bleeding • Thrombocytopenia with LTU
Eptifibatide (Integrilin)	• **A:** IV • **E:** Parent drug and products of its breakdown excreted in urine	• Reversible blockade of glycoprotein IIb/IIIa receptor		
Ticlopidine (Ticlid)	• **A:** PO; well absorbed • **M:** Hepatic metabolism • **E:** Metabolites excreted in urine and feces	• Irreversible inhibition of ADP-mediated platelet aggregation	• Less effective than aspirin but useful in patients who are intolerant to aspirin • Prevention of TIAs and ischemic strokes	• Excessive bleeding • Nausea • Dyspepsia • Diarrhea • Severe neutropenia (rare) • Thrombotic thrombocytopenic purpura
Clopidogrel (Plavix)	• **A:** PO • **M:** Hepatic metabolism to active metabolites • **E:** Metabolites excreted in feces and urine		• Prevention of ischemic events	• Fewer side effects than ticlopidine • Thrombotic thrombocytopenic purpura

DRUGS USED TO FACILITATE CLOTTING

Drug	Pharmacokinetics	Mechanism of Action	Clinical Uses	Side Effects
Fat Soluble Vitamin				
Vitamin K	• A: PO or IV	• Supplementation of naturally occurring endogenous substance responsible for carboxylation of coagulation factors VII, IX, X, and II	• Treatment of vitamin K–deficient states as is seen in newborns and the elderly • Reversal of warfarin overdose	• Rapid IV infusion can cause dyspnea, chest and back pain, or death
Endogenous or Recombinant Plasma Components				
Clotting factors	• A: IV	• Supplementation of endogenous plasma clotting factors	• Treatment of hemophilia • Treatment of bleeding diathesis	• Once associated with hepatitis B and C and HIV transmission • Still carry some risk of blood-borne pathogens
Antiplasmin Drug				
Aminocaproic acid (Amicar)	• A: IV or PO • E: Renal excretion of unchanged drug	• Inhibits fibrinolysis via inhibition of plasminogen activation	• Treatment of acute bleeding episodes in hemophilia and other bleeding disorders • Prophylaxis for rebleeding from intracranial aneurysms	• Intravascular thrombosis • Hypotension • Myopathy • Abdominal discomfort • Diarrhea

CHAPTER 7
RESPIRATORY DRUGS

TERMS TO LEARN

Antitussive	Drug that relieves or prevents cough.
Antihistamine	Drug that counteracts histamine; can be divided into two groups: those that block H_1 histamine receptors and those that block H_2 receptors.
Area Postrema	A region of the brain located in the medulla at the base of the 4th ventricle; location of the chemoreceptive trigger zone where vomiting is triggered.
Churg-Strauss Syndrome	Vasculitis of the small arteries and veins; characterized by extravascular necrotizing granulomas; typically seen in patients with asthma or an allergy history.
Decongestant	Drug that reduces congestion or swelling.
Expectorant	Drug that promotes ejection of mucus or exudate from respiratory tract.

I. Cold Medications

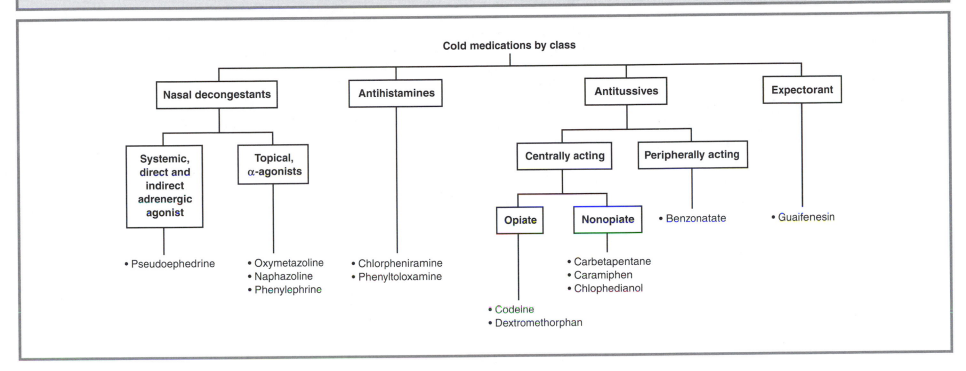

COLD MEDICATIONS: DRUG FACTS

Drug	Mechanism of Action	Clinical Uses	Drawbacks and Side Effects
Systemic Decongestants			
Pseudoephedrine (Sudafed)	• Vasoconstriction of blood vessels in nasal mucosa	• Vasoconstriction effect on respiratory vasculature causes decrease in nasal congestion	• Contraindicated in patients with hypertension, past MI, or hyperthyroidism because it increases blood pressure
Topical Decongestants			
Oxymetazoline (Afrin, Dristan)	• Vasoconstriction in nasal mucosa leads to decreased inflammation of mucosa and decreased nasal stuffiness		• Rebound congestion
Naphazoline (Privine)			• Irregular heartbeat
Phenylephrine (Neo-Synephrine)			• Headache • Dizziness • Tremor
Antihistamines (See Chapter 12 for Complete List of H$_1$ Blockers)			
Chlorpheniramine (Chlor-Trimeton)	• Prevent histamine from acting on H$_1$ receptors		• Cause paralysis of the mucociliary escalator
Phenyltoloxamine (Comhist-LA)	• Prevention of stimulation of sneeze reflex receptors by histamine • Antimuscarinic effects decrease bronchial secretions and increase bronchial dilation		• Anticholinergic side effects • Sedation

Antitussives			
Codeine	• Suppression of coughing by action on the μ receptors in the area postrema (cough center)	• Cough suppressant • Analgesic	• Nausea and vomiting • Bitter taste • Action on μ receptors in GI decreases motility leading to constipation • Highly addictive due to ability to produce euphoric state • Causes the release of histamine, which leads to bronchoconstriction, vasodilation, and increased mucus production (counteracts action of other medications)
Dextromethorphan (Robitussin-DM)		• Cough suppressant • Does not produce euphoria at therapeutic doses • Produces less constipation than codeine	• Histamine release (less than codeine) • Not as effective as codeine • Overdose can produce hallucinatory effect
Carbetapentane (Rynatuss) Caramiphen (Tuss-Ade) Chlophedianol (Ulone)		• Used in low doses in pediatric population where opiates and dextromethorphan are contraindicated for cough control	• Anticholinergic side effects

Continued

COLD MEDICATIONS: DRUG FACTS (Continued)

Drug	Mechanism of Action	Clinical Uses	Drawbacks and Side Effects
Benzonatate (Tessalon)	• Decreases sensitivity of peripheral cough receptors	• Cough suppressant	• Confusion • Hypersensitivity reactions • Convulsions (with overdose)
Expectorant			
Guaifenesin/glyceryl guaiacolate (Robitussin A-C Syrup, Entex)	• Activates irritant receptors in the GI tract, which cause impulses to be sent to the CNS producing parasympathetic stimulation in both the GI and respiratory tracts • Leads to increased production of less viscous mucus • Increases activity of mucociliary escalator	• Prevention of the formation of mucous plugs in patients with CF or COPD • Produces more voluminous, less dense mucus, which promotes cleaning of the airway	• GI upset

II. Asthma Drugs

CLASSIFICATION OF ASTHMA DRUGS

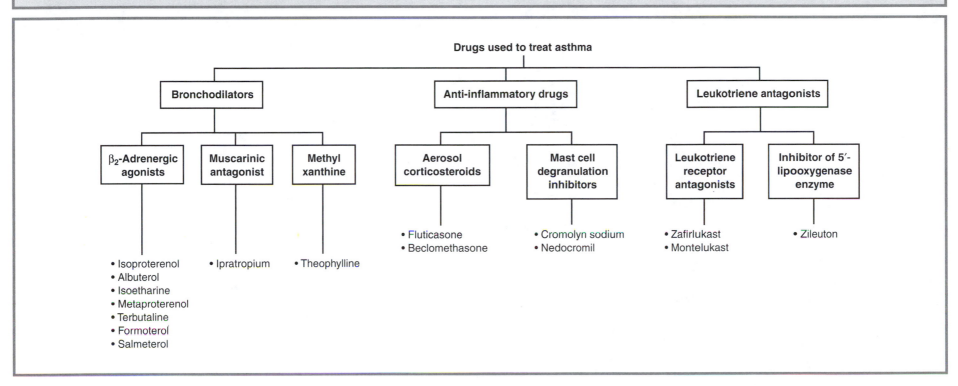

Drugs used to treat asthma

Bronchodilators

β₂-Adrenergic agonists
- Isoproterenol
- Albuterol
- Isoetharine
- Metaproterenol
- Terbutaline
- Formoterol
- Salmeterol

Muscarinic antagonist
- Ipratropium

Methyl xanthine
- Theophylline

Anti-inflammatory drugs

Aerosol corticosteroids
- Fluticasone
- Beclomethasone

Mast cell degranulation inhibitors
- Cromolyn sodium
- Nedocromil

Leukotriene antagonists

Leukotriene receptor antagonists
- Zafirlukast
- Montelukast

Inhibitor of 5′-lipooxygenase enzyme
- Zileuton

β_2-ADRENERGIC AGONISTS

Drug	Pharmacokinetics	Mechanism of Action	Clinical Uses	Side Effects
Nonselective β_2-Agonist				
Isoproterenol (Isuprel)	• **A:** Inhalation and IV • **DOA and OOA:** Short • **M:** Local tissue metabolism; hepatic metabolism following IV administration • **E:** Parent drug and metabolites excreted in urine	• β_2-Stimulation causes increased AC, which causes an increase in cAMP in smooth muscle leading to bronchodilation	• Asthma • Other uses include treatment of hyperkalemia (cause K^+ to enter cells) and relaxation of uterine contractions	• Tolerance due to down-regulated receptors • Some β_1-adrenergic actions are seen, which lead to decreased BP and increased HR • Tremor due to receptor stimulation on skeletal muscle • Nervousness and excitation • Weakness • Dizziness • Flushing of the face or skin • Nausea and vomiting
β_2-Adrenergic Agonist				
Albuterol (Proventil, Ventolin)	• **A:** inhalation and PO • **DOA and OOA:** Short • **M:** Hepatic metabolism • **E:** Parent drug and metabolites excreted in urine			
Isoetharine	• **A:** Inhalation • **DOA and OOA:** Short • **M:** COMT metabolism then hepatic metabolism • **E:** Parent drug and metabolites excreted in urine			
Metaproterenol (Alupent, Metaprel)	• **A:** Inhalation and PO • **DOA and OOA:** Short • **M:** Extensive first-pass hepatic metabolism • **E:** Parent drug and metabolites excreted in urine			

Terbutaline (Brethine)	• **A:** Inhalation, PO, SC, IV • **DOA and OOA:** Short • **M:** Partial hepatic metabolism • **E:** Parent drug and metabolites excreted in urine
Formoterol (Foradil)	• **A:** Inhalation • **DOA and OOA:** Short • **M:** Hepatic metabolism • **E:** Parent drug and metabolites excreted in urine and feces
Salmeterol (Serevent)	• **A:** Inhalation • **DOA:** Long • **M:** Hepatic metabolism • **E:** Metabolites excreted in feces

NON–β_2-ADRENERGIC AGONISTS

Drug	Pharmacokinetics	Mechanism of Action	Clinical Uses	Side Effects
Muscarinic Antagonist				
Ipratropium (Atrovent)	• **A:** Inhaled (highly ionized in alveoli so not well absorbed) and nasal • **M:** Hepatic metabolism • **E:** Parent drug and metabolites excreted in urine and feces	• Prevents bronchoconstriction mediated by vagal muscarinic discharge	• Asthma	• Limited systemic absorption reduces anticholinergic side effects
Methyl Xanthine				
Theophylline (Elixophyllin, Slo-Phyllin, Uniphyl, Theo-Dur, Theo-24)	• **A:** PO and IV • **M:** Hepatic metabolism • **E:** Parent drug and metabolites excreted in urine	• Inhibits PDE and therefore increases cAMP levels • Increased cAMP in mast cells causes decreased degranulation	• Bronchodilator in COPD patients (once used to treat asthma)	• GI irritant • Inhibits PDE in skeletal muscle causing force of contraction of accessory muscles to be increased • CNS stimulant (can produce seizures) • Enters myocardium and produces β-receptor responses (increased ionotropy and chronotropy)
Aerosol Corticosteroids				
Fluticasone (Flovent)	• **A:** Inhalation • **M:** Absorbed portion metabolized in liver • **E:** Majority of metabolites excreted in feces; remainder in urine	• Vasoconstriction and anti-inflammatory properties via unknown mechanisms (possibly via actions on mast cells)	• Asthma (maintain patency of airway with onset of late inflammation) • Control acute and late inflammatory phases	• Churg-Strauss syndrome • Rhinitis
Beclomethasone (Vancenase)	• **A:** Intranasal (pharmacokinetics not well defined for intranasal administration)			• Nasal burning • Headache

Mast Cell Degranulation Inhibitor

Cromolyn sodium (Intal, Nasalcrom) Nedocromil (Tilade)	• **A:** PO and inhaled; local effects only due to poor absorption • **E:** Unchanged in bile and urine	• Prevent release of leukotrienes and histamine from mast cells	• Prophylaxis for bronchial asthma • Prophylaxis for allergic rhinitis • Blocks both early- and late-phase responses	• Can cause coughs because of irritation due to aerosolized administration

Leukotriene Receptor Antagonist

Zafirlukast (Accolate)	• **A:** PO • **M:** Hepatic metabolism by P450 enzymes • **E:** Majority of metabolites excreted in feces; remainder in urine	• LTD_4- and LTE_4-receptor blockers	• Prophylaxis for acute bronchospastic attacks	• Headache • Nausea • Infection
Montelukast (Singulair)				• Headache • Abdominal pain • Churg-Strauss syndrome

Inhibitor of 5′-Lipooxygenase Enzyme

Zileuton (Zyflo)	• **A:** PO • **M:** Hepatic metabolism • **E:** Metabolites excreted in urine	• Prevents formation of leukotrienes	• Dyspepsia • Diarrhea • Headache

POSSIBLE MECHANISMS OF ASTHMA DRUGS

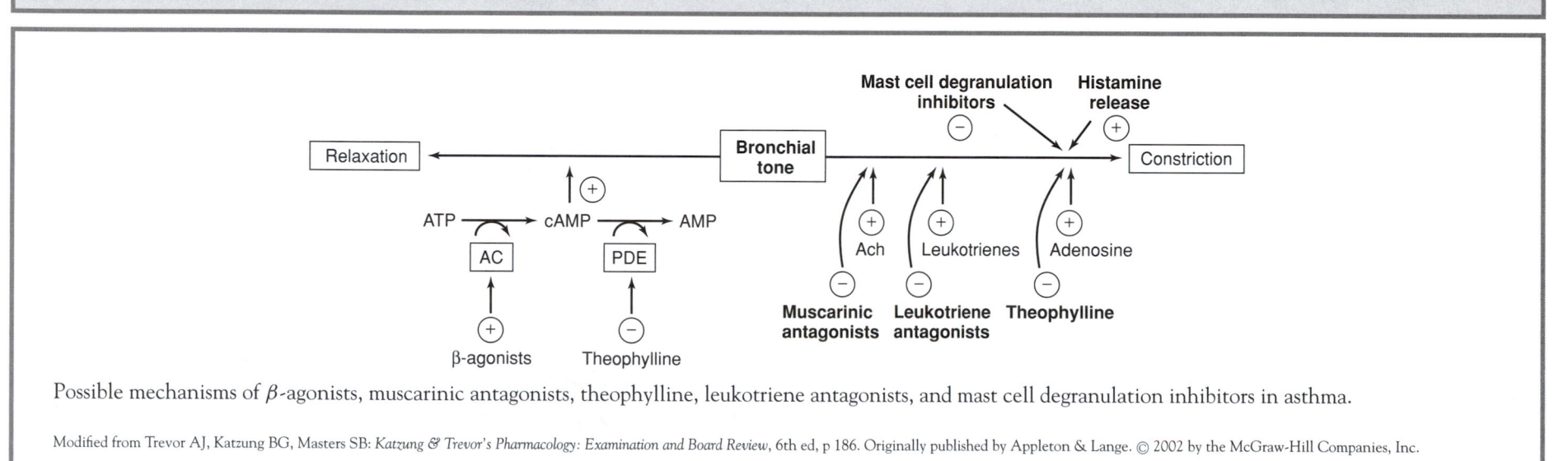

Possible mechanisms of β-agonists, muscarinic antagonists, theophylline, leukotriene antagonists, and mast cell degranulation inhibitors in asthma.

Modified from Trevor AJ, Katzung BG, Masters SB: *Katzung & Trevor's Pharmacology: Examination and Board Review*, 6th ed, p 186. Originally published by Appleton & Lange. © 2002 by the McGraw-Hill Companies, Inc.

CHAPTER 8
GASTROINTESTINAL DRUGS

TERMS TO LEARN

Anticholelithic	Drug that can dissolve gallstones.
Antiemetic	Prevents or alleviates nausea and vomiting.
Blood Dyscrasias	Disorders of the cellular elements of the blood.
Chemoreceptor Trigger Zone	Part of the brain that induces vomiting; located in the area postrema at the base of the 4th ventricle outside the BBB; it is exposed to medications/toxins in blood and CSF.
Gastroparesis	Paralysis of the stomach.
Gynecomastia	Growth of breast tissue in males.
Zollinger-Ellison Syndrome	Associated with gastrin secreting tumors causing hypergastrinemia and acid hypersecretion; 90% of these patients have PUD.

I. H₂ Blockers

H₂-RECEPTOR ANTAGONISTS

Drug	Pharmacokinetics	Mechanism of Action	Clinical Uses	Side Effects
Cimetidine (Tagamet)	• **A:** PO, IM, IV; oral availability 40–50% • $t_{1/2}$: 1.5–2.3 hours • **M:** Hepatic metabolism • **E:** Metabolites and parent drug excreted in urine	• Decreases gastric acid secretion via competitive inhibition of H₂ receptors	• PUD (heals gastric and duodenal ulcers and prevents their recurrence) • Esophagitis • Zollinger-Ellison syndrome • Prophylaxis for NSAID-induced duodenal ulcers • Prophylaxis for stress-induced ulcers	• Blood dyscrasias • CNS confusion (slurred speech and confusion in the elderly) • Gynecomastia with LTU due to antiandrogenic action (blocks the production and release of testosterone; can be used by transsexuals for breast development) • Inhibits cytochrome P450 system, leading to drug interactions
Famotidine (Pepcid)	• **A:** PO, IM, IV; oral availability 37–45% • $t_{1/2}$: 2.5–4 hours • **M:** Small amount of hepatic metabolism • **E:** Most eliminated in urine			• Hepatic abnormalities (hepatitis with famotidine, LFT abnormalities with nizatidine and reversible hepatitis with ranitidine) • Headache • Dizziness • Diarrhea ☞ Cimetidine's side effects all contain **C**'s. Other **H₂** blockers have 2 **H**'s and 2 **D**'s.
Nizatidine (Axid)	• **A:** PO; oral availability 75–100% • $t_{1/2}$: 1.1–1.6 hours • **M:** Hepatic metabolism • **E:** In urine (small amount in feces)			
Ranitidine (Zantac)	• **A:** PO, IM, IV; oral availability 30–88% • $t_{1/2}$: 1.6–2.4 hours • **M:** Extensive first-pass metabolism • **E:** In urine and feces			

II. Antacids and Proton Pump Inhibitors

ANTACIDS: DRUG FACTS

Drug	Pharmacokinetics	Mechanism of Action	Clinical Uses	Side Effects
Aluminum hydroxide	• **A:** PO; not significantly absorbed • **E:** In feces; absorbed portion excreted in urine	• Weak bases that react with gastric acid to produce salt and water	• Symptomatic relief of GERD, PUD, esophagitis, and gastric hyperacidity	• Constipation • Hypokalemia
Calcium carbonate	• **A:** PO; 30% absorbed (vitamin D–dependent) • **E:** Absorbed portion excreted in urine	• Increase gastric pH • Pepsin inactivated when gastric pH is >4	• Safe for use during pregnancy • Better at healing duodenal ulcers than gastric ulcers	• Hypercalcemia • Metabolic alkalosis • Hypokalemia
Magnesium hydroxide	• **A:** PO; not significantly absorbed • **E:** Absorbed portion excreted in urine			• Strong laxative effect
Sodium bicarbonate	• **A:** PO • **E:** Absorbed portion excreted in urine			• Metabolic alkalosis

PROTON PUMP INHIBITORS: DRUG FACTS

Drug	Pharmacokinetics	Mechanism of Action	Clinical Uses	Side Effects
Esomeprazole (Nexium) Omeprazole (Prilosec) Lansoprazole (Prevacid) Pantoprazole (Protonix) Rabeprazole (Aciphex) ☞ **Proton pump inhibitors all end in prazole.**	• **A:** PO • **M:** Hepatic metabolism by P450 enzymes • **E:** Metabolites excreted in urine and feces	• Irreversibly inhibits acid secretion (new enzymes required for acid secretion to resume) • Activated when secreted into acidic environment of stomach • Coating on tablet is digested in duodenum and drug is released and absorbed	• GERD • PUD • Esophagitis • NSAID-induced ulcers • Zollinger-Ellison syndrome	• Diarrhea • Nausea • Constipation • Headache • Dizziness

III. Other Medications for Treating GI Diseases

OTHER AGENTS FOR GI DISEASES: DRUG FACTS

Drug	Class	Pharmacokinetics	Mechanism of Action	Clinical Uses	Side Effects
Atropine (Sal-Tropine)	• Muscarinic antagonist	• **A:** IM, IV, PO, SC, and inhaled • **M:** Hepatic metabolism • **E:** Parent drug and metabolites excreted in urine (small amounts exhaled and excreted in feces)	• Reduces basal acid secretion 40–50%	• Antisecretory agent • Used in conjunction with H_2 blockers or in refractory cases of PUD • When H_2 antagonists are not effective	• Anticholinergic side effects
Bismuth Subsalicylate (Pepto Bismol)	• Colloidal bismuth compound	• **A:** PO • **M:** Metabolized in the GI tract • **E:** Metabolites excreted in urine and feces	• Mucosal protective agent • Increases mucus secretion, which forms a barrier to acid diffusion to the ulcer • Causes detachment and lysis of *Helicobacter pylori*	• PUD • Diarrhea	• Encephalopathy with LTU or overdose
Misoprostol (Cytotec)	• Prostaglandin E_1 analogue	• **A:** PO • **M:** Extensive first-pass hepatic metabolism • **E:** Majority of parent drug and metabolites excreted in urine; remainder in feces	• Mucosal protective agent • Suppresses gastric acid secretion	• Prophylaxis for NSAID-induced ulcers • PUD	• Diarrhea • Abdominal pain

Sucralfate (Carafate)	• Aluminum sucrose sulfate	• **A:** PO; minimal absorption • **E:** Unchanged in feces	• Mucosal protective agent • Polymerizing gel (polymerizes at pH ≤4) that adheres to bare ulcer crater and protects it to allow healing)	• PUD	• Few side effects due to minimal absorption
Ondansetron (Zofran)	• 5-HT₃ antagonist	• **A:** PO, IM, IV • **M:** Hepatic metabolism • **E:** Metabolites excreted in urine	• Blocks 5-HT₃ receptors both centrally and peripherally • May act to reduce the action of 5-HT in the chemoreceptor trigger zone (CTZ)	• Antiemetic	• Diarrhea
Prochlorperazine (Compazine)	• Phenothiazine	• **A:** PO, IM, IV, and rectal	• Blocks DA receptors in the CTZ	• Antiemetic	• EPS with large doses • Sedation
Chenodiol (Chenix)	• Bile acid derivatives	• **A:** PO • **M:** Hepatic metabolism • **E:** Metabolites excreted in feces	• Inhibits formation of gallstones by reducing the secretion of bile acids from the liver	• Anticholelithic	• Diarrhea
Ursodiol (Actigall)			• Inhibits formation of gallstones via unknown mechanism • May act through inhibition of hepatic cholesterol synthesis and reduced cholesterol absorption allowing cholesterol to be solubilized from existing gallstones		• Back pain • Diarrhea
Metoclopramide (Reglan)	• DA blocker	• **A:** PO, IM, IV • **M:** Hepatic metabolism • **E:** Parent drug and metabolites excreted in urine	• Stimulate gastric motility by inhibiting DA-induced gastric smooth muscle relaxation (allows for unopposed cholinergic tone)	• Gastroparesis	• Diarrhea • Drowsiness • EPS • Restlessness

COMBINATION THERAPIES

Therapy	Clinical Use	Protocol	Complications
H₂ receptor antagonist with antibiotics	• Treatment of peptic ulcers	• Ranitidine with amoxicillin and metronidazole	• Negligible
Bismuth-based triple therapy	• Treatment of duodenal or gastric ulcers with confirmed H Pylori infection	• Tritec (bismuth citrate with ranitidine) plus two antibiotics such as: — clarithromycin and metronidazole — tetracycline and metronidazole — clarithromycin and amoxicillin OR • Helidac (bismuth subsalicylate), H₂ receptor antagonist plus tetracycline and metronidazole	• Triple therapy **must** be given because using an antibiotic alone to eradicate H Pylori infection leads to the rapid development of drug resistance. • High incidence of side effects such as diarrhea, nausea and vomiting, abdominal discomfort, and headache make compliance a problem.
Proton pump inhibitors with two antibiotics	• Treatment of duodenal or gastric ulcers with confirmed H Pylori infection	• Omeprazole or lansoprazole plus two antibiotics such as: — clarithromycin and metronidazole — tetracycline and metronidazole — clarithromycin and amoxicillin	• Proton pump inhibitors have a bacteriostatic effect on H Pylori (H Pylori does not become resistant to amoxicillin) • Combination therapy **must** be given because using antisecretory therapy alone will not eradicate H Pylori infection. • These combination therapies can lead to such side effects as diarrhea, nausea, vomiting, abdominal discomfort, and headaches.

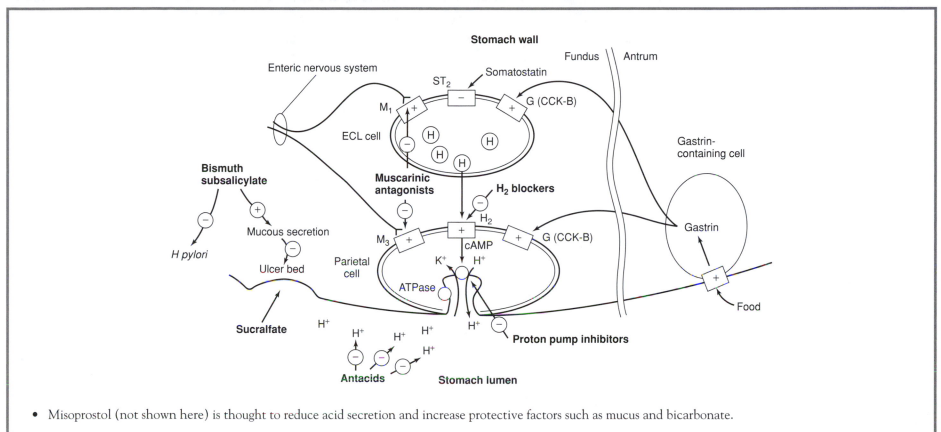

- Misoprostol (not shown here) is thought to reduce acid secretion and increase protective factors such as mucus and bicarbonate.

CHAPTER 9

DRUGS AFFECTING THE ENDOCRINE SYSTEM

TERMS TO LEARN

Acromegaly	Syndrome associated with excessive levels of growth hormone after puberty; symptoms include thickened skin, vocal hoarseness, joint pain, insulin resistance, hypertension, and cardiovascular disease.
Asthenia	Debility or weakness.
Carcinoid Syndrome	Symptoms associated with excessive levels of serotonin secreted by carcinoid tumors; symptoms include facial swelling, diarrhea, bronchial spasm, tachycardia, hypotension, and right-sided valvular disease.
Central Precocious Puberty	Early onset of puberty due to activation of the gonadotropins leading to maturation of the gonads; this early gonadal maturation leads to early secretion of sex hormones and, therefore, early onset of secondary sexual characteristics in adolescents.
Craniosynostosis	Premature closure of the cranial sutures.
Cushing's Disease	Disease associated with excessive glucocorticoid levels most commonly caused by an adrenal cortical adenoma; symptoms include fat redistribution with a characteristic buffalo hump, thin extremities, hypertension, hirsutism, infertility, and amenorrhea.
Diabetes Insipidis	Syndrome due to insufficient levels of ADH (central) or decreased renal response to ADH (peripheral); symptoms resemble the excessive thirst and urination associated with diabetes mellitus.
Endometriosis	Growth of cells of the uterine lining outside of the uterus; symptoms include pelvic pain and infertility.
Hyperprolactinemia	Syndrome associated with excessive levels of prolactin; symptoms include infertility, amenorrhea, galactorrhea, and mastodynia.
Hypogonadotropic Hypogonadism	Inadequate function of the gonads due to insufficient secretion of pituitary gonadotropins.
Kaposi's Sarcoma	Rare skin malignancy characterized by soft blue-black plaques and is typically seen in elderly and immunosuppressed patients; it is caused by human herpes virus 8.
Oligospermia	Low sperm count.

SIADH	Syndrome of inappropriate ADH; numerous causes include trauma, tumors, endocrine disorders, and drugs; excessive levels of ADH lead to hypernatremia.
Steatorrhea	Large amounts of fat in the feces.
Uterine Fibroids	Benign smooth muscle tumors; their growth is related to estrogen.
Virilization	Acquisition of adult male characteristics in women or prepubescent males.

I. Hypothalamic and Pituitary Hormones

HYPOTHALAMIC-PITUITARY HORMONAL AXIS

Hypothalamic Hormone	Pituitary Hormone	Target Organ	Target Organ Hormone
Hypothalamic hormones regulate the release of anterior pituitary hormones. Oxytocin and vasopressin are produced in the posterior pituitary (an outgrowth of the hypothalamus) where they are released into general circulation. All the endocrine agents listed below are peptides, except for prolactin-inhibiting hormone.			
Growth hormone-releasing hormone (GHRH)	Growth hormone (GH)	Liver	Somatomedins
Somatostatin[a]			
Thyrotropin-releasing hormone (TRH)	Thyroid-stimulating hormone (TSH)	Thyroid	Thyroxine, triiodothyronine
Corticotropin-releasing hormone (CRH)	Adrenocorticotropic hormone (ACTH)	Adrenal cortex	Glucocorticoids, mineralocorticoids, androgens
Gonadotropin-releasing hormone (GnRH or LHRH)	Follicle-stimulating hormone (FSH) Luteinizing hormone (LH)	Gonads	Estrogen, progesterone, testosterone
Prolactin-releasing hormone (PRH)	Prolactin (PRL)	Lymphocytes	Lymphokines
Prolactin-inhibiting hormone (PIH, dopamine)		Breast	—
Oxytocin		Smooth muscle, especially uterus	—
Vasopressin		Renal tubule, smooth muscle	—

[a]Inhibits GH and TSH release. Also found in GI tissues; inhibits release of gastrin, glucagon, and insulin.

Modified from Trevor AJ, Katzung BG, Masters SB: *Katzung & Trevor's Pharmacology Examination and Board Review*, 6th ed. Originally published by Appleton & Lange. © 2002 by the McGraw-Hill Companies, Inc.

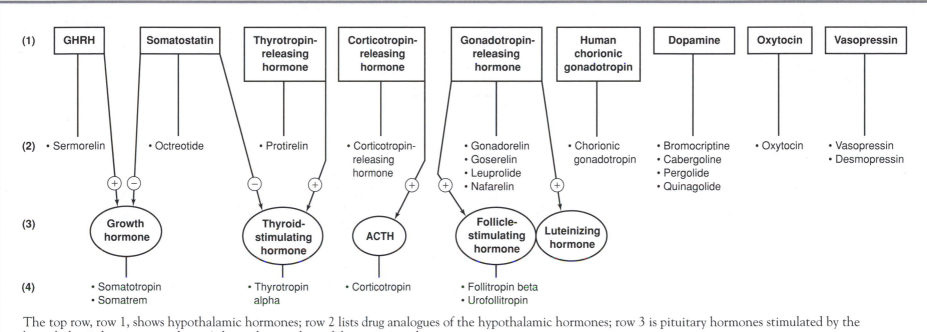

The top row, row 1, shows hypothalamic hormones; row 2 lists drug analogues of the hypothalamic hormones; row 3 is pituitary hormones stimulated by the hypothalamic hormones; and row 4 shows drug analogs of those pituitary hormones.

EXOGENOUS HYPOTHALAMIC AND PITUITARY HORMONES

Drug	Mimicked Hormones	Route of Administration	Clinical Uses	Side Effects
Octreotide (Sandostatin)	• Somatostatin analog	• IM, IV, or SC	• Symptomatic reduction of syndromes from hormone-secreting tumors including acromegaly, carcinoid syndrome, gastrinoma, glucagonoma • Also effective for controlling acute bleeding from esophageal varices	• Nausea • Abdominal cramps • Flatulence • Steatorrhea
Sermorelin (Geref)	• GHRH	• IV or SC	• Treatment of GH-deficient states with intact pituitary responsiveness	• Headache • Facial flushing • Injection site pain • Nausea
Somatotropin (Genotropin, Humatrope, and others)	• Recombinant growth hormones	• IM or SC	• Treatment of GH-deficient states • Improves growth in children with failure to thrive due to chronic renal failure caused by HIV infection	• Arthralgia • Gynecomastia • Hypothyroidism • Intracranial hypertension • Pancreatitis • Peripheral edema • Scoliosis due to rapid growth
Somatrem (Protropin)		• IM or SC	• Treatment of GH-deficient states	
Protirelin (Thypinone, Relefact TRH)	• Thyrotropin-releasing hormone	• IV	• Diagnostic tool for hypothalamic-pituitary-thyroid axis function	• Blood pressure instability • Flushing • Light-headedness • Metallic taste • Nausea • Urge to urinate

Thyrotropin Alpha (Thyrogen)	• Recombinant thyroid-stimulating hormone	• IM	• Detection of metastatic differentiated thyroid carcinoma	• Nausea • Headache • Asthenia
Corticotropin-releasing hormone	• Exogenous CRH	• IM, IV, and SC	• Diagnostic tool for the differentiation of Cushing's disease from ectopic ACTH secretion	• Facial flushing (transient) • Dyspnea
Corticotropin (ACTH, Acthar, and others)	• Exogenous corticotropin	• IM or SC	• Diagnostic tool to assess adrenocorticol responsiveness	• Rare with doses used for diagnostic evaluations
Gonadorelin (Lutrepulse, Factrel)	• Exogenous gonadotropin-releasing hormone	• IV or SC	• Diagnostic tool to test pituitary luteinizing hormone responsiveness • Female infertility • Male infertility caused by hypothalamic GnRH deficiency	• Headache • Flushing and light-headedness • Nausea
Goserelin (Zoladex)		• SC implant	• Treatment of endometriosis, breast cancer, and dysfunctional uterine bleeding • Treatment of prostate cancer	In women: • Depression • Diminished libido
Leuprolide (Lupron)		• IM and SC	• Treatment of endometriosis and uterine fibroids • Treatment of prostate cancer • Treatment of central precocious puberty	• Headache • Hot flashes and sweats • Vaginal dryness
Nafarelin (Synarel)		• Nasal	• Treatment of endometriosis • Treatment of central precocious puberty	In men: • Asthenia • Diminished libido • Edema • Gynecomastia • Hot flashes and sweats

Continued

EXOGENOUS HYPOTHALAMIC AND PITUITARY HORMONES (Continued)

Drug	Mimicked Hormones	Route of Administration	Clinical Uses	Side Effects
Follitropin Beta (Follistim) Urofollitropin (Fertinex, Metrodin)	• Exogenous follicle-stimulating hormone	• IM and SC	• Treatment of infertility (stimulate ovarian follicle development in women and spermatogenesis in men)	• Gynecomastia • Multiple births • Uncomplicated ovarian enlargement
Chorionic Gonadotropin (Profasi, Pregnyl)	• Exogenous human chorionic gonadotropin	• IM	• Used as a substitute for LH • Diagnostic differentiation between retained or retracted undescended testes • Diagnostic differentiation between constitutional delay and hypogonadotropic hypogonadism in adolescents with delayed puberty • Induction of ovulation in women with hypogonadotropic hypogonadism or as part of in vitro fertilization • Regression of AIDS-related Kaposi's sarcoma with injection directly into lesion	• Depression • Edema • Gynecomastia • Headache • Precocious puberty
Bromocriptine (Parlodel) Cabergoline (Dostinex) Pergolide (Permax) Quinagolide (Norprolac)	• Dopamine agonists	• PO or intravaginal • PO or intravaginal • PO	• Treatment of prolactin-secreting adenomas • Symptomatic relief of hyperprolactinemia • Treatment of acromegaly • Treatment of Parkinson's disease (bromocriptine and pergolide)	• Headache • Fatigue • Light-headedness • Nausea • Orthostatic hypotension • Psychiatric disturbances

Oxytocin (Pitocin, Syntocinon)	• Exogenous oxytocin	• IV or nasal	• Diagnostic evaluation of placental circulatory reserve • Induction or augmentation of labor • Control of postpartum uterine hemorrhage • Treatment of impaired milk ejection	• Maternal death due to hypertensive episodes or uterine rupture
Vasopressin (Pitressin Synthetic)	• Exogenous vasopressin or antidiuretic hormone	• IM, IV, SC, or intranasal	• Treatment of diabetes insipidus • Treatment of esophageal variceal or colonic diverticular bleeding	• Abdominal cramps • Agitation • Headache • Hyponatremic convulsions with overdose • Nausea • Vasoconstriction
Desmopressin (DDAVP, Stimate)		• PO, SC, IV, and intranasal	• Treatment of diabetes insipidus • Treatment of nocturnal enuresis by decreasing nocturnal urine production	• Abdominal cramps • Agitation • Headache • Hyponatremic convulsions with overdose • Nausea

II. Glucocorticoids and Mineralocorticoids

EXOGENOUS GLUCOCORTICOIDS

Drug	Pharmacokinetics				Clinical Uses	Side Effects
	Route of Administration	$t_{1/2}$	Anti-inflammatory Potency*	Mineralocorticoid Potency*		
Hydrocortisone (Cortef, Anusol HC, Westcort)	IM, IV, SC, PO, intra-articular, intralesional	12 hours	1.0	1.0	• Skin and eye irritations • Prevention of transplant rejection	• Adrenal insufficiency (requires tapering dosage to avoid this effect) • Behavioral disturbances • Glucose intolerance • Impaired wound healing • Increased intracranial pressure with high doses • Osteoporosis • Peptic ulcers
Prednisone (Deltasone, Meticorten)	PO	12–24 hours	4.0	0.8	• Severe allergic reactions • Prevention of transplant rejections	
Triamcinolone (Aristocort, Aristospan, Nasacort)	PO, IM, intralesional, intra-articular, or inhaled	24 hours	5.0	0	• Skin irritations	
Dexamethasone (Decadron, Dexasone)	PO, IM, IV, intralesional, intra-articular	36 hours	30.0	0	• Severe allergic reactions and asthma	

*Hydrocortisone is the basis of the potency for the rest of the glucocorticocoids.

MINERALOCORTICOIDS: AGONIST AND ANTAGONIST

Drug	Pharmacokinetics	Mechanism of Action	Clinical Uses	Side Effects
Mineralocorticoid Agonist				
Fludrocorticosone (Florinef)	• **A:** PO • **M:** Hepatic and renal metabolism • **E:** Metabolites excreted in urine	• Adrenal corticoid steroid with high mineralocorticoid and moderate glucocorticoid activity • Acts at distal tubule to increase K^+ and H^+ excretion leading to increased Na^+ and H_2O retention	• Treatment of adrenocortical insufficiency • Treatment of type IV RTA associated with hyporeninemic hypoaldosterone • Treatment of idiopathic orthostatic hypotension	• Anaphylaxis • CHF • Edema • Hypertension • Hypokalemic alkalosis • Increased ICP • Mental disturbances • Osteoporosis • Pancreatitis
Mineralocorticoid Antagonists				
Metyrapone (Metopirone)	• **A:** PO; well absorbed • **M:** Hepatic metabolism • **E:** Parent drug and metabolites excreted in urine	• Inhibits enzymatic 11-β hydroxylation of desoxycorticosone leads to decreased production of cortisol and aldosterone; should result in increased CRH and ACTH, which will lead to accumulation of cortisol and aldosterone precursors • Metabolites of these precursors can be measured in urine	• Diagnosis of adrenal insufficiency • Diagnosis and short-term treatment of Cushing's syndrome	• Allergic skin rash • Bone marrow depression • Headache • Nausea
Spironolactone (Aldactone)	• **A:** PO • **M:** Metabolized to active metabolites • **E:** Majority of metabolites excreted in urine; remaining are excreted in feces	• Blocks the effects of aldosterone in the collecting duct leading to Na^+ loss and K^+ retention • Inhibits the activity of aldosterone at the collecting duct	• Hyperaldosterone states • Combined with thiazide diuretics to treat hypertension	• Hyperkalemia • Gynecomastia • Antiandrogenic effects

III. Thyroid Drugs

MEDICATIONS FOR TREATING THYROID CONDITIONS

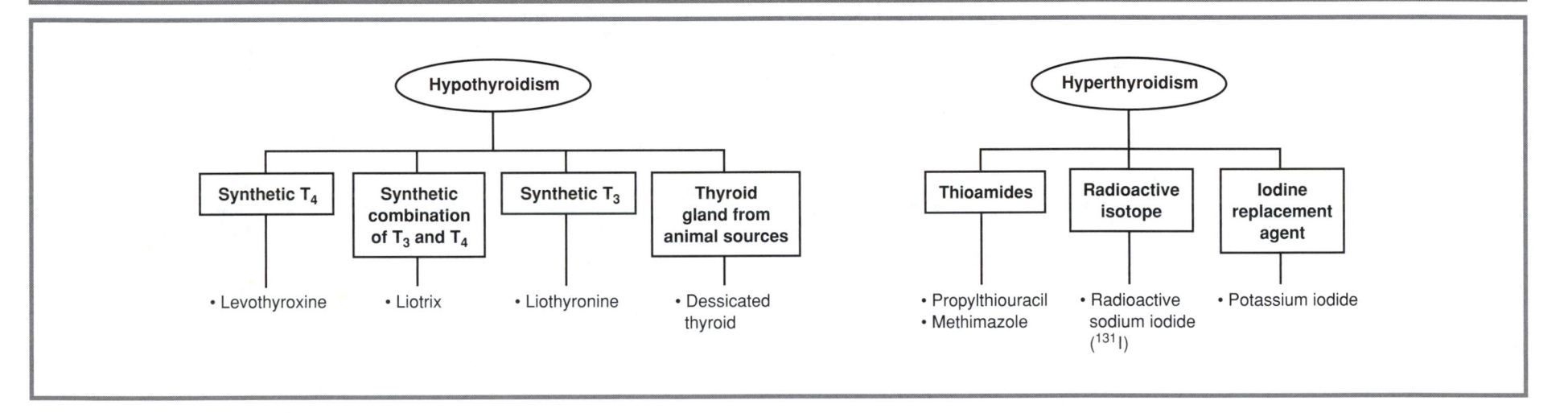

MEDICATIONS FOR TREATING HYPOTHYROIDISM

Drug	Class	Pharmacokinetics	Mechanism of Action	Clinical Uses and General Information	Side Effects
Levothyroxine (Levothroid, Levoxyl, Synthroid)	• Synthetic form of T_4	• **A:** PO, IM or IV • **M:** Hepatic metabolism • **E:** Metabolites excreted in feces	• Same mechanism of action as endogenous thyroid hormones	• Hypothyroidism • IV preparation is useful for emergency situations	• Craniosynostosis with iatrogenic hyperthyroidism in pregnant women • Rash • Urticaria
Liothyronine (Cytomel, Triostat)	• Synthetic form of T_3	• **A:** PO and IM • **M:** Hepatic metabolism • **E:** Metabolites excreted in feces		• Hypothyroidism • IV preparation is useful for emergency situations • More potent than levothyronine	• Allergic skin reactions • Arrhythmias • Tachycardia
Liotrix (Thyrolar)	• Synthetic combination of T_3 and T_4 in 1:4 ratio	• **A:** PO • **M:** Hepatic metabolism • **E:** Metabolites excreted in feces		• Hypothyroidism	• Hyperthyroidism due to iatrogenic overdose
Desiccated thyroid (Armour Thyroid, Thyroid Strong, Thyrar, S-P-T)	• Thyroid gland from animal sources	• **A:** PO • **M:** Hepatic metabolism • **E:** Metabolites excreted in feces		• Hypothyroidism • Inexpensive • Natural ratio T_3 and T_4	

MEDICATIONS FOR TREATING HYPERTHYROIDISM

Drug	Class	Pharmacokinetics	Mechanism of Action	Clinical Uses and General Information	Side Effects
Propylthiouracil (PTU)	Thioamides	• **A:** PO • **M:** Hepatic metabolism • **E:** Parent drug and metabolites excreted in urine	• Inhibits thyroidal peroxidase	• Hyperthyroidism • The thyroid often resumes its normal function after about 2 years of therapy • Safer than methimazole for use during pregnancy • Also inhibits peripheral conversion of T_4 to T_3	• Blood dyscrasias • Nausea • Nephritis • Pruritus • Rash
Methimazole (Tapazole)		• **A:** PO • **E:** In urine		• Hyperthyroidism • The thyroid often resumes its normal function after about 2 years of therapy	
Radioactive sodium iodide (^{131}I, Iodotope)	Radioactive isotope	• **A:** PO • **E:** In urine (small amounts excreted in feces and saliva)	• Taken up by gland to destroy tissue internally	• Hyperthyroidism • Thyroid carcinoma	• Hyperthyroidism or hypothyroidism • Leukopenia • Thrombocytopenia
Potassium iodide (SSKI, Lugol's Solution, Pima, Iodo-niacin)	Iodine replacement agent	• **A:** PO	• Acts as a competitive inhibitor of the radioactive isotopes of iodine • Decreases the activity of an overactive thyroid gland	• Hyperthyroidism • Prophylactic treatment of individuals near radioactive accidents	• Angioedema • Arthralgia • Diarrhea • Nausea

IV. Medications Affecting Calcium Levels

MEDICATIONS AFFECTING CALCIUM LEVELS: DRUG FACTS				

Drug	Pharmacokinetics	Mechanism of Action	Clinical Uses	Side Effects
Serum Estrogen Receptor Modulators				
Tamoxifen (Nolvadex)	• **A:** PO • **M:** Hepatic metabolism • **E:** Majority of metabolites excreted in feces; remainder in urine	• Estrogen antagonist on breast tissue and in CNS • Estrogen agonist on endometrium, bones, and lipids • Precise MOA unknown	• Prophylaxis and treatment of postmenopausal osteoporosis	• Endometrial hyperplasia/carcinoma • Headache • Hepatotoxicity • Hot flashes • Nausea
Raloxifene (Evista)				• Chest pain • Cystitis • Leg cramping • Peripheral edema
Bisphosphonates				
Alendronate (Fosamax)	• **A:** PO, poorly absorbed; etidronate also available in IV form • **E:** Unchanged in urine; unabsorbed portion excreted unchanged in feces	• Bind to bone hydroxyapatite and inhibit osteoclast activity at the cellular level	• Treatment and prevention of osteoporosis in women • Osteoporosis in men • Corticosteroid-induced osteoporosis • Paget's disease	• Esophagitis • GERD

Continued

MEDICATIONS AFFECTING CALCIUM LEVELS: DRUG FACTS (Continued)

Drug	Pharmacokinetics	Mechanism of Action	Clinical Uses	Side Effects
Etidronate (Didronel)			• Paget's disease • Hypercalcemia associated with malignancy • Treatment and prophylaxis for heterotropic ossification following hip replacements or spinal cord injuries	• Allergic reactions (angioedema, skin rash, etc.) • Bone pain • Diarrhea • Nausea • Osteomalacia
Pamidronate (Aredia)	• **A:** IV • **E:** Unchanged in urine		• Paget's disease • Hypercalcemia associated with malignancy • Adjunctive treatment for osteolytic bone metastases	• Hypocalcemia • Leukopenia • Lymphopenia
Risedronate (Actonel)	• **A:** PO • **E:** Unchanged in urine; unabsorbed portion excreted unchanged in feces		• Treatment and prevention of osteoporosis in women • Osteoporosis in men • Corticosteroid-induced osteoporosis • Treatment of Paget's disease	• Abdominal pain • Allergic reactions (angioedema, skin rash, etc.) • Bone pain • Diarrhea

Thiazide Diuretic

Hydrochlorothiazide (HCTZ)	• **A:** PO • **E:** Unchanged in urine	• Reduces renal Ca^{2+} excretion • May increase the effectiveness of PTH in stimulating Ca^{2+} reabsorption by the renal tubules	• Hypercalciuria • Nephrolithiasis secondary to hypercalciuria	• Increases in serum Ca^{2+}, Mg^{2+}, glucose, lipids, uric acids • Decreases in serum K^+ and Na^+ • Metabolic alkalosis • Muscle weakness • Pancreatitis • Vasodilation

Antineoplastic Agent

Plicamycin (Mithracin)	• **A:** IV • **E:** In urine	• Reduces serum Ca^{2+} via unknown mechanism (possibly via inhibition of DNA-dependent synthesis that renders the osteoclast unable to respond to PTH)	• Hypercalcemia associated with malignancy • Paget's disease • Testicular CA • Limited clinical use because of severe side effect profile	• Hemorrhage • Hepatotoxicity • Nephrotoxicity • Thrombocytopenia

Dental Prophylaxis

Sodium fluoride (Fluoritab)	• **A:** PO	• Accumulates in bone where it stabilizes the hydroxyapatite crystal	• Prophylaxis for dental caries • Under investigation as a possible treatment of osteoporosis	• Overdose discolors teeth

CLINICAL USES OF MEDICATIONS THAT AFFECT CALCIUM LEVELS

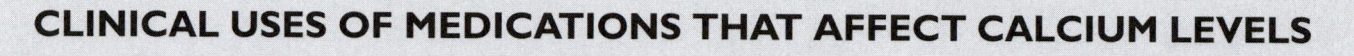

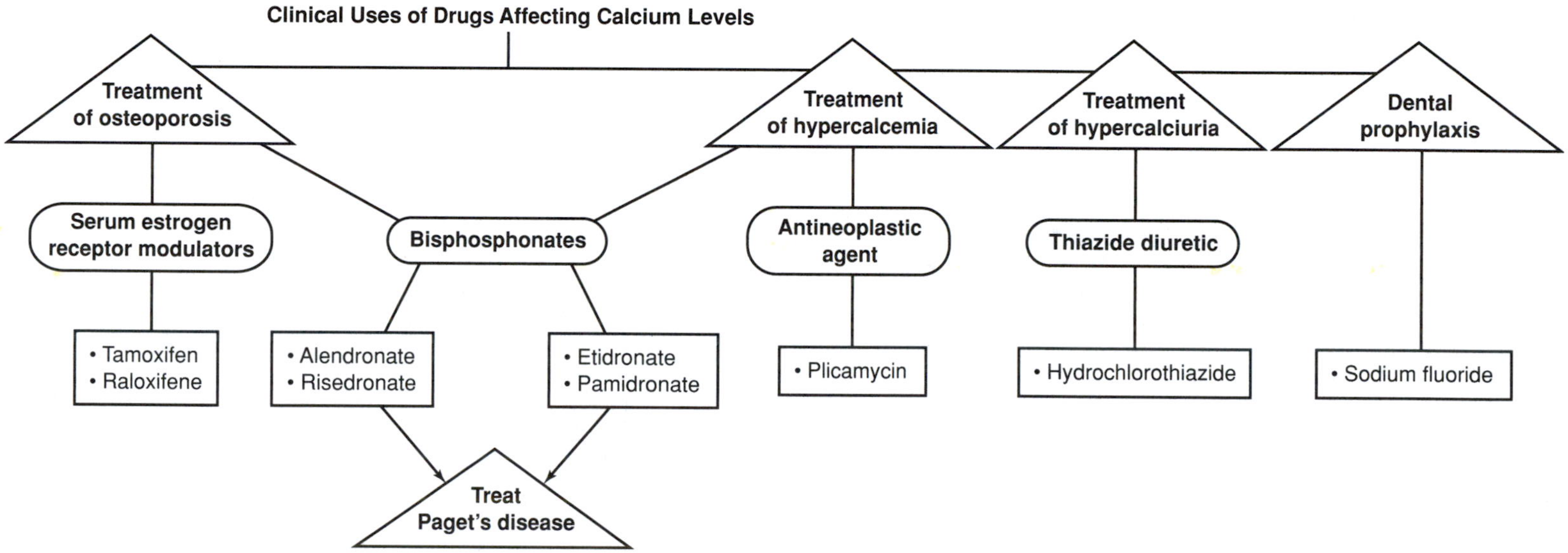

Clinical Uses of Drugs Affecting Calcium Levels

Treatment of osteoporosis

Treatment of hypercalcemia

Treatment of hypercalciuria

Dental prophylaxis

Serum estrogen receptor modulators

Bisphosphonates

Antineoplastic agent

Thiazide diuretic

- Tamoxifen
- Raloxifene

- Alendronate
- Risedronate

- Etidronate
- Pamidronate

- Plicamycin

- Hydrochlorothiazide

- Sodium fluoride

Treat Paget's disease

V. Medications for Managing Diabetes

TYPES OF INSULIN

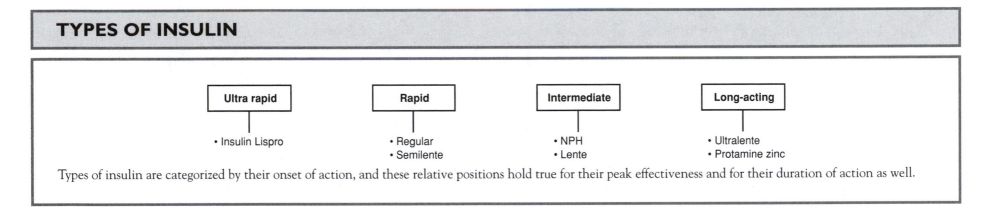

Ultra rapid	Rapid	Intermediate	Long-acting
• Insulin Lispro	• Regular • Semilente	• NPH • Lente	• Ultralente • Protamine zinc

Types of insulin are categorized by their onset of action, and these relative positions hold true for their peak effectiveness and for their duration of action as well.

INSULIN: DRUG FACTS

Drug	Appearance	Pharmacokinetics				Clinical Uses	Side Effects
		Route of Administration	Onset	Peak	Duration		
Insulin Lispro	• Clear	IV and SC	20 min	30 min	3–4 hours	• Suitable for use immediately before meals	• Hypoglycemia • Allergies due to noninsulin components of the preparations
Regular		SC	30 min	1–3 hours	5–8 hours	• Available for IV administration in emergency situations • Available for continuous subcutaneous infusion • Combined with NPH to form Novolin 70/30 or Humulin 70/30 or 50/50	
Semilente	• Cloudy		30–60 min	2–8 hours	12–16 hours	• Used in combination with Ultralente to form Lente	
NPH			1–2 hours	6–12 hours	18–24 hours	• Combined with regular to form Novolin 70/30 or Humulin 70/30 or 50/50	
Lente						• Mixture of 30% Semilente and 70% Ultralente	
Ultralente			4–6 hours	8–16 hours	20–36 hours	• Provides a basal insulin level that lasts 24 hours	
Protamine Zinc			4–6 hours	14–20 hours	24–36 hours	• Often combined in a regimen including injections of regular insulin for optimal control	

CLASSIFICATION OF ORAL DIABETIC DRUGS

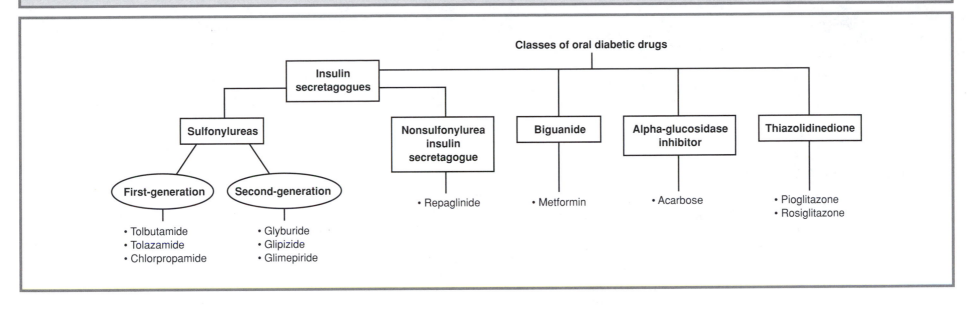

9. Drugs Affecting the Endocrine System

ORAL DIABETIC DRUGS: SULFONYLUREAS

Drug	Pharmacokinetics	Mechanism of Action	Characteristics	Side Effects
First-Generation Sulfonylureas				
Tolbutamide (Orinase)	• **DOA:** 6–12 hours • **M:** Hepatic metabolism • **E:** Metabolites excreted in urine and feces	• Bind to ATP-sensitive K^+ channels to block the efflux of K^+ resulting in membrane depolarization thus increasing the Ca^{2+} entering the cell thereby increasing the insulin release • Potentiate exocytosis of insulin containing granules by direct binding to intracellular binding sites • Increase action of insulin on target tissues by increasing the number of insulin receptors	• Weakest of the sulfonylureas • Safest of the class for elderly patients • Only useful when some endogenous insulin is being produced • Works best with restricted calorie intake and weight reduction	• Headaches • Heartburn • Hypoglycemia • Nausea • Rash
Tolazamide (Tolinase)	• **DOA:** 10–14 hours • **M:** Hepatic metabolism to active metabolites • **E:** Parent drug and metabolites excreted in urine		• Higher potency and slower onset of action than tolbutamide • Only useful when some endogenous insulin is being produced • Works best with restricted calorie intake and weight reduction	• Hypoglycemia • GI symptoms (nausea, vomiting, diarrhea) • CNS symptoms (weakness, fatigue, lethargy) • Hematologic effects (thrombocytopenia, leukopenia, agranulocytosis)
Chlorpropamide (Diabinese)	• **DOA:** Up to 60 hours • **M:** Hepatic metabolism to active metabolites • **E:** Parent drug and metabolites excreted in urine		• Only useful when some endogenous insulin is being produced • Works best with restricted calorie intake and weight reduction	• Hematologic toxicity • Jaundice • Prolonged hypoglycemia is more common than with other sulfonylureas

Second-Generation Sulfonylureas

Glyburide (Diabeta, Glynase, Micronase, Pres-Tab)	• **DOA:** 10–24 hours • **M:** Hepatic metabolism • **E:** Parent drug and metabolites excreted in urine and feces	• Allow for once a day dosing • 100 times more potent than first-generation	• Cholestatic jaundice • Hypoglycemia (more pronounced with glyburide and glipizide) • Weight gain • SIADH • GI symptoms (nausea, vomiting, diarrhea) • Hematologic effects (thrombocytopenia, leukopenia, agranulocytosis)
Glipizide (Glucotrol)	• **DOA:** 10–24 hours • **M:** Hepatic metabolism to active metabolites • **E:** Majority of parent drug and metabolites excreted in urine; remainder in feces		
Glimepiride (Amaryl)	• **DOA:** 12–24 hours • **M:** Hepatic metabolism • **E:** Metabolites excreted in urine		

ORAL DIABETIC DRUGS: NONSULFONYLUREAS

Drug	Pharmacokinetics	Mechanism of Action	Characteristics	Side Effects
Nonsulfonylurea Insulin Secretagogue				
Repaglinide (Prandin)	• **DOA:** 1–3 hours • **M:** Hepatic metabolism by P450 enzymes • **E:** Majority of metabolites excreted in urine	• Closes an ATP-dependent K⁺ channel to block the efflux of K⁺ resulting in membrane depolarization thus increasing the Ca^{2+} entering the cell thereby increasing the insulin release	• Effect on blood glucose is similar to sulfonylurea • Lacks sulfur in its structure; therefore useful in patients who cannot take sulfonylureas because of allergy to sulfur • Works well with metformin	• Arthralgias • Diarrhea • Headache • Hypoglycemia • Nausea • Paresthesia
Biguanide				
Metformin (Glucophage)	• **DOA:** 10–12 hours • **E:** Unchanged in the urine	• Increases insulin receptor binding in liver, adipose, and muscle for increased glucose uptake • Inhibits hepatic gluconeogenesis	• Useful in patients with refractory obesity with ineffective insulin action • Used in combination with sulfonylureas	• Diarrhea • Nausea • Abdominal discomfort
α-Glucosidase Inhibitor				
Acarbose (Precose)	• **DOA:** 3–4 hours • **M:** Metabolized by intestinal flora • **E:** Unabsorbed portion excreted in feces; absorbed metabolites excreted in urine	• Slows carbohydrate digestion and absorption time to prevent exaggerated postprandial rise in blood glucose	• Only decreases postprandial hyperglycemia by 30–50% • Does not cause hypoglycemia • Due to decreased blood glucose rise; insulin release is also diminished • Reduces nonenzymatic glycation of proteins • Reduced glucose levels improves overall glucose control and insulin sensitivity	• Abdominal pain • Diarrhea • Flatulence • Jaundice

Thiazolidinediones

Pioglitazone (Actos)	• **DOA:** 15–24 hours • **M:** Hepatic metabolism by P450 enzymes • **E:** Majority of parent drug and metabolites excreted in feces; remainder of metabolites excreted in urine	• Increase glucose uptake in muscle and adipose • Decrease insulin resistance and lower hepatic gluconeogenesis • Exact mechanism not well understood	• Less effective than sulfonylureas or biguanides • Useful for monotherapy or combined with a biguanide • Cause a redistribution of body fat with a decrease in central obesity	• Edema • Headache • Hypoglycemia • Upper respiratory tract infections
Rosiglitazone (Avandia)	• **DOA:** >24 hours • **M:** Hepatic metabolism by P450 enzymes • **E:** Metabolites excreted in urine and feces			

VI. Drugs Affecting Reproductive Hormones

CLINICAL USES FOR VARIOUS ESTROGEN PREPARATIONS

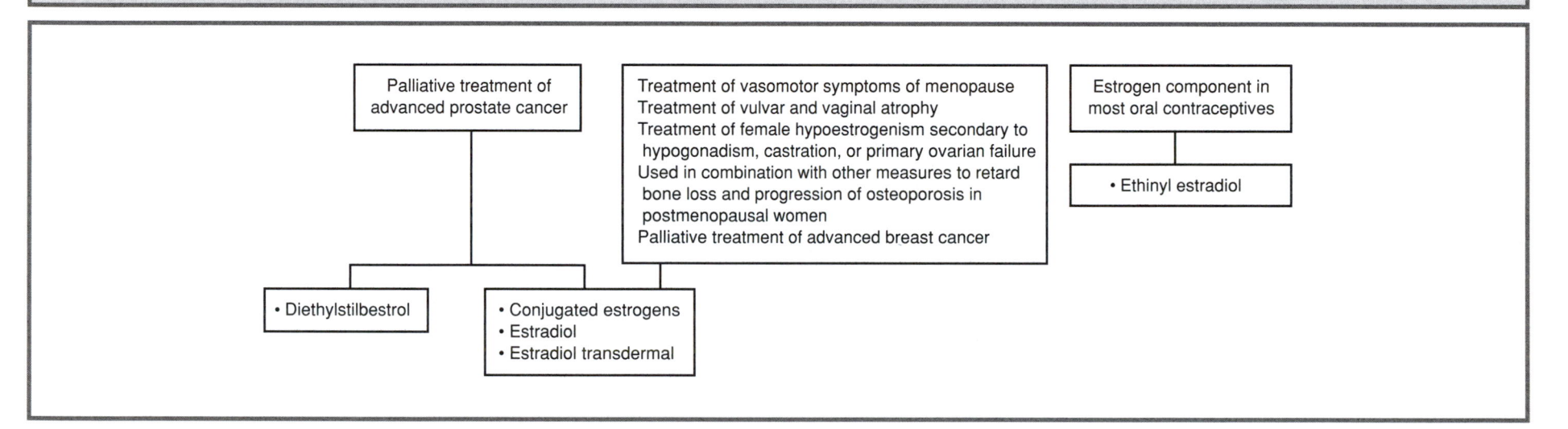

Palliative treatment of advanced prostate cancer

- Diethylstilbestrol
- Conjugated estrogens
- Estradiol
- Estradiol transdermal

Treatment of vasomotor symptoms of menopause
Treatment of vulvar and vaginal atrophy
Treatment of female hypoestrogenism secondary to hypogonadism, castration, or primary ovarian failure
Used in combination with other measures to retard bone loss and progression of osteoporosis in postmenopausal women
Palliative treatment of advanced breast cancer

Estrogen component in most oral contraceptives

- Ethinyl estradiol

ESTROGEN PREPARATIONS: DRUG FACTS

Drug	Route of Administration	Clinical Uses and General Information	Drawbacks and Side Effects
Conjugated estrogens (Premarin)	• PO, IM, IV, and vaginal	• Treatment of vasomotor symptoms of menopause • Treatment of vulvar and vaginal atrophy	• Nausea and vomiting • Edema
Estradiol (Estrace and others)	• PO, IM, and vaginal	• Treatment of female hypoestrogenism secondary to hypogonadism, castration, or primary ovarian failure • Used in combination with other therapeutic measures to retard bone loss and progression of osteoporosis in postmenopausal women • Palliative treatment of advanced breast CA • Palliative treatment of advanced prostate CA	• Headache • Hepatic neoplasias • Breast tenderness • Venous thrombosis/thromboembolism • Breakthrough bleeding • Unopposed estrogen causes endometrial hyperplasia and possible endometrial carcinoma (should be administered with progesterone)
Estradiol transdermal (Climara, Estraderm, Fempatch, and others)	• Transdermal patches	• Uses same as above • Achieves a higher physiologic E_2/E_1 ratio and avoids first-pass metabolism by the liver • Eliminates wide fluctuations in serum levels of the drug	
Ethinyl estradiol (Estinyl)	• PO	• Estrogen component in most oral contraceptives	
Diethylstilbestrol/ DES (Stilphostrol)	• IV and PO	• Palliative treatment of advanced prostate CA	• Same as above • Increased incidence of adenocarcinoma of the vagina in female offspring of patients who have taken this drug

ANTIESTROGEN DRUGS

Drug	Pharmacokinetics	Mechanism of Action	Clinical Uses and General Information	Drawbacks and Side Effects
Clomiphene (Clomid, Serophene, Milophene)	• **A:** PO • **M:** Hepatic metabolism • **E:** Majority of metabolites excreted in feces; remainder in urine	• Estrogen receptor agonist in CNS and GU organs (endometrium, vagina, cervix, and ovary) • Causes preovulatory gonadotropin surge	• Fertility drug that induces ovulation in anovulatory conditions • Blocks estrogen's inhibitory effect on the hypothalamus and pituitary leading to increased FSH/LH levels • Increased LH/FSH levels produce ovulation	• Allergic skin reactions • Constipation • Depression • Headache • Hot flashes • Ovarian enlargement • Reversible hair loss • Multiple births
Tamoxifen (Nolvadex)		• Estrogen antagonist in breast tissue and CNS • Estrogen agonist on endometrium, bone, and lipids	• Used to treat estrogen receptor–negative breast CA in premenopausal women • Can be used prophylactically in women with a history of breast CA • Positive effects on bone density and lipid profile	• Endometrial hyperplasia/carcinoma • Headache • Hepatotoxicity • Hot flashes • Nausea
Raloxifene (Evista)		• Mixed estrogen agonist/antagonist • Estrogen agonist at estrogen receptors on bone, CVS, and CNS	• Prophylaxis and treatment of postmenopausal osteoporosis • Lowers LDL levels • Does not cause endometrial hyperplasia associated with tamoxifen	• Chest pain • Cystitis • Leg cramping • Peripheral edema

COMBINATIONS OF ESTROGEN AND PROGESTERONE

Numerous hormone replacement therapy and contraception preparations are estrogen and progesterone combinations. This combination avoids the endometrial hyperplasia and possible carcinoma associated with unopposed estrogen.

Drug	Route of Administration	Formula	Clinical Uses	Side Effects
Conjugated estrogen and medroxyprogesterone (Premphase)	• PO	• 14 days of estrogen followed by 14 days of estrogen and progesterone	• Treatment of estrogen-deficient states	• Amenorrhea (with constant progesterone)
Conjugated estrogen and medroxyprogesterone (Prempro)	• PO	• Constant dose of estrogen and progesterone		• Breast tumors • Changes in uterine bleeding • Gallbladder obstruction • Hepatitis • Pancreatitis • Skin rash
Ethinyl estradiol and norethindrone (Brevicon, Modicon)	• PO	• Constant dose of estrogen and progesterone	• Contraception	• Breakthrough bleeding • Headache
Ethinyl estradiol and norethindrone (Ortho-Novum 10/11)	• PO	• Constant dose of estrogen with 2 doses of progesterone (second dose is larger)		• Mastalgia • Nausea • Thromboembolic disease
Ethinyl estradiol and norgestimate (Ortho-Tri-Cylcen)	• PO	• Constant dose of estrogen with 3 increasing doses of progesterone each week		• Weight gain
Ethinyl estradiol and norethindrone (Ortho-Novum 7/7/7)	• PO			

PROGESTERONE PREPARATIONS

Note that the four progesterone preparations used as contraceptives contain either "nor" or "progesterone" in their names. Megestrol is not used as a contraceptive.

Drug	Route of Administration	Clinical Uses	Side Effects
Levonorgestrel (Norplant)	• SC implant	• Contraceptive (implant provides 5 years of contraception) • Emergency postcoital contraception	• Abdominal pain • Amenorrhea • Breast pain • Hot flushes • Irregular or prolonged periods of uterine bleeding • Leukorrhea • Libido changes • Thromboembolic disease • Weight gain
Medroxyprogesterone (Depo Provera, Cycrin, and others)	• PO and IM	• Contraceptive (IM injection provides 3 months of contraception) • Treatment of abnormal uterine bleeding • Adjunctive and palliative therapy for the treatment of advanced endometrial and renal CA • Treatment of paraphilia in males	
Megestrol (Megace)	• PO	• Palliative therapy for the treatment of advanced endometrial and breast CA • Treatment of AIDS-related anorexia and cachexia	
Norethindrone Minipill (Micronor, Overette, Aygestin)	• PO	• Contraceptive (daily PO dosing) • Treatment of abnormal uterine bleeding caused by hormonal imbalance • Treatment of endometriosis	
Progesterone intrauterine device (Progestasert)	• Intrauterine device	• Contraceptive (provides 1 year of contraception)	• Similar side effects as above • Cervical or uterine trauma

ANTIPROGESTERONE DRUG

Drug	Pharmacokinetics	Mechanism of Action	Clinical Uses	Side Effects
Mifepristone (RU-486, Mifeprex, Mifegyne)	• **A:** PO • **M:** Metabolized by hepatic P450 enzymes • **E:** Metabolites excreted in urine and feces	• Competitive inhibitor at progesterone and glucocorticoid receptors	• Abortifacient agent • Potential use in the treatment of Cushing's disease due to glucocorticoid receptor–blocking quality • Emergency postcoital contraceptive agent • Fewer side effects as a postcoital contraceptive than the high dose estrogen "morning after pill"	• Abdominal pain • Anemia • Diarrhea • Dizziness • Nausea • Vomiting

TESTOSTERONE PREPARATIONS

Drug	Route of Administration	Clinical Uses	Side Effects
Fluoxymesterone (Halotestin)	• PO	• Treatment of testosterone-deficient states • Palliative treatment of androgen-responsive advanced breast CA in women • Used in combination with ethinyl estradiol for short-term management of vasomotor symptoms associated with menopause	• Acne • Cholestatic hepatitis • Headache • Hypercalcemia due to osteolysis • Gynecomastia • Edema • Mood changes • Nausea • Oligospermia • Virilization
Methyltestosterone (Android, Testred, Virilon, and others)	• PO and sublingual		
Testosterone cypionate (Depo-Testosterone and others)	• IM	• Treatment of testosterone-deficient states	
Testosterone enanthate (Delatestryl and others)	• IM	• Treatment of testosterone-deficient states	
Testosterone propionate (Androlan, Testex)	• IM	• Palliative treatment of androgen-responsive advanced breast CA in women	

GENERAL THERAPEUTIC USES OF TESTOSTERONE

- Primary hypogonadism (post orchidectomy, bilateral testicular torsion, etc.)
- Hypogonadotropic hypogonadism (GnRH deficiency, pituitary/hypothalamic injury from tumors, trauma, or radiation)
- Androgen replacement therapy for Leydig cell deficiency
- Promoting muscle mass in acute illness, severe trauma, and other malnourished states due to chronic illness
- Palliative treatment of androgen-responsive advanced carcinoma of the breast in women

ANTIANDROGEN DRUGS

Drug	Class	Pharmacokinetics	Mechanism of Action	Clinical Uses	Side Effects
Leuprolide (Lupron)	Gondadotropin-releasing hormone analog (GnRH agonists)	• **A:** IM or SC • **M:** Metabolized to smaller peptides (probably in hypothalamus and pituitary) • **E:** Small amounts of metabolites excreted in urine	• Causes down-regulation of the receptors in the pituitary leading to decreased hormonal output	• Treatment of BPH • Treatment of prostate CA • Other uses include treatment of precocious puberty, hirsutism, endometriosis, dysmenorrhea, and uterine leiomyoma	• Hot flashes in men and women • Amenorrhea • Initial prostate cancer flare (severe pain associated with initial increase in serum testosterone)
Finasteride (Proscar, Propecia)	5 α-reductase inhibitor	• **A:** PO • **M:** Hepatic metabolism • **E:** Metabolites excreted in feces and urine	• Inhibits the enzyme responsible for the conversion of testosterone to its more potent form dihydrotestosterone	• Treatment of BPH • Lower doses are useful for reduction of hair loss in men	• Gynecomastia • Hypersensitivity reactions
Flutamide (Eulexin, Etaconil)	Nonsteroidal antiandrogen	• **A:** PO • **M:** Hepatic metabolism • **E:** Parent drug and metabolites excreted in urine	• Competitive antagonist at androgen receptor	• Used in combination with a GnRH analog in the treatment of prostate CA • Can prevent the "flare response" with the initiation of treatment	• Hepatotoxicity (reversible)

Continued

ANTIANDROGEN DRUGS (Continued)

Drug	Class	Pharmacokinetics	Mechanism of Action	Clinical Uses	Side Effects
Spironolactone (Aldactone)	17α-hydroxylase inhibitor	• **A:** PO • **M:** Metabolized to active metabolites • **E:** Majority of metabolites are excreted in urine; remaining in feces	• Competitive inhibitor of dihydrotestosterone in target tissues • Inhibits 17α-hydroxylase activity, thereby decreasing testosterone production	• Treatment of hirsutism in women	• Hypersensitivity reactions • Gastritis • Gynecomastia • Impotence
Cyproterone (Androcur)	Steroidal antiandrogen	• **A:** PO and IM • **M:** Hepatic metabolism • **E:** Metabolites excreted in feces and urine	• Competitive antagonist at androgen receptor	• Treatment of hirsutism • Treatment of excessive sex drive in men • Palliative treatment of advanced prostate CA	• Hepatotoxicity • Galactorrhea • Gynecomastia • Impotence
Ketoconazole (Nizoral)	Antifungal agent	• **A:** PO and topical • **M:** Hepatic metabolism • **E:** Parent drug and metabolites excreted in feces and urine	• Inhibits gonadal and adrenal steroid synthesis	• Treatment of advanced prostate CA • Treatment of hirsutism	• Gynecomastia • Hepatotoxicity • Impotence

292 | 9. Drugs Affecting the Endocrine System

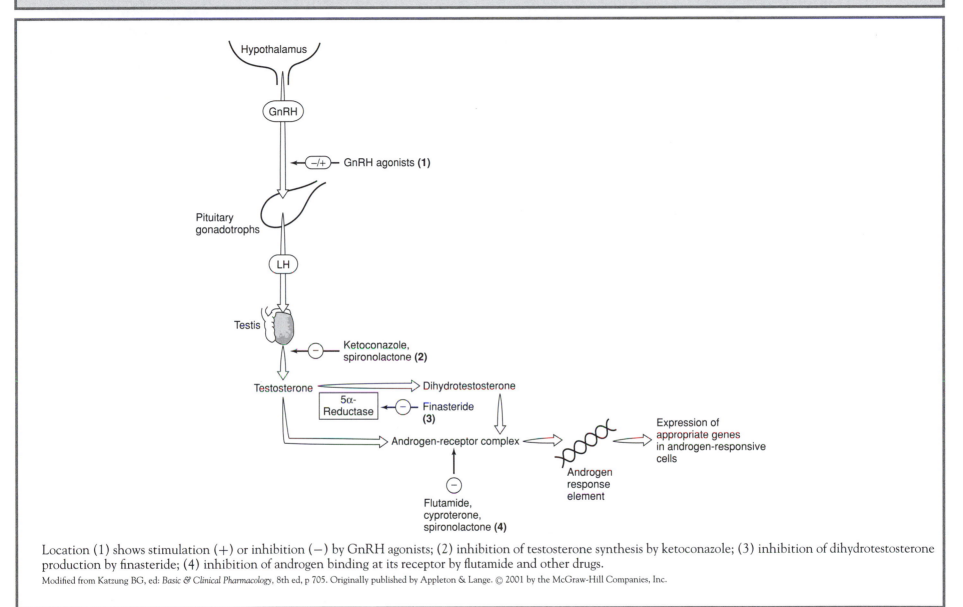

Location (1) shows stimulation (+) or inhibition (−) by GnRH agonists; (2) inhibition of testosterone synthesis by ketoconazole; (3) inhibition of dihydrotestosterone production by finasteride; (4) inhibition of androgen binding at its receptor by flutamide and other drugs.

Modified from Katzung BG, ed: *Basic & Clinical Pharmacology*, 8th ed, p 705. Originally published by Appleton & Lange. © 2001 by the McGraw-Hill Companies, Inc.

CHAPTER 10
ONCOLOGIC DRUGS

I. ACTION OF ONCOLOGIC MEDICATIONS

Oncologic Drugs by Mechanism of Action

Phases of the Cell Cycle

II. ALKYLATING DRUGS

Alkylating Drug Facts

III. ANTIMETABOLITES

Antimetabolites: Pyrimidine, Purine, and Folic Acid Antagonists

IV. ANTITUMOR ANTIBIOTICS

Action of Antitumor Antibiotics

Antitumor Antibiotics: Cell Cycle-Specific and Cell Cycle-Nonspecific Drugs

V. PLANT ALKALOIDS

Plant Alkaloids by Action and Class

Plant Alkaloids: Drug Facts

VI. HORMONAL ANTICANCER DRUGS

Classification of Hormonal Anticancer Drugs

Hormonal Anticancer Drug Facts

VII. CHEMOTHERAPEUTIC DRUGS

Miscellaneous Chemotherapeutics: Drug Facts

Chemotherapeutics: Monoclonal Antibodies

TERMS TO LEARN

Chronic Myelogenous Leukemia	Bone marrow malignancy involving myeloid cells; it is typically seen in older patients and is associated with poor prognosis.
Ewing's Sarcoma	Malignancy of the bone; seen in young boys.
Gestational Trophoblastic Neoplasms	Group of malignancies stemming from fetal or placental tissue.
Giant Cell Tumors	Benign bone tumor.
Hodgkin's Lymphoma	Malignancy of the lymph nodes; bimodal age distribution (seen in young and old men); associated with a good prognosis with chemotherapy.
Multiple Myeloma	Malignancy of plasma cells; it is characterized by bone pain, "punched out" lytic lesion of the bone, hypercalcemia, and Bence Jones proteinuria.
Neuroblastoma	Most common extracranial solid tumor of childhood; malignancy that arises from the neural crest cells that tends to occur in the abdomen and thorax; it secretes catecholamines.
Non-Hodgkin's Lymphoma	Malignancy of the lymph nodes; more likely to have extranodal primaries (ie, stomach or thyroid) than Hodgkins lymphoma; it is associated with a poorer prognosis than Hodgkins lymphoma.
Wilms' Tumor	Renal malignancy seen in children; it is associated with hemihypertrophy of the body.

I. Action of Oncologic Medications

ONCOLOGIC DRUGS BY MECHANISM OF ACTION*

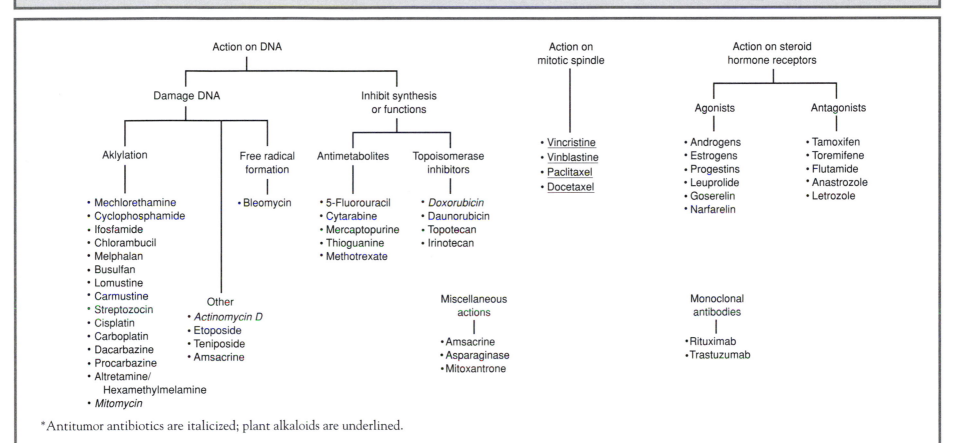

Action on DNA

Damage DNA

Inhibit synthesis or functions

Aklylation

Free radical formation

Antimetabolites

Topoisomerase inhibitors

Action on mitotic spindle

• Vincristine
• Vinblastine
• Paclitaxel
• Docetaxel

Action on steroid hormone receptors

Agonists

Antagonists

- Mechlorethamine
- Cyclophosphamide
- Ifosfamide
- Chlorambucil
- Melphalan
- Busulfan
- Lomustine
- Carmustine
- Streptozocin
- Cisplatin
- Carboplatin
- Dacarbazine
- Procarbazine
- Altretamine/ Hexamethylmelamine
- *Mitomycin*

• Bleomycin

- 5-Fluorouracil
- Cytarabine
- Mercaptopurine
- Thioguanine
- Methotrexate

- *Doxorubicin*
- *Daunorubicin*
- Topotecan
- Irinotecan

Other
- *Actinomycin D*
- Etoposide
- Teniposide
- Amsacrine

Miscellaneous actions
- Amsacrine
- Asparaginase
- Mitoxantrone

- Androgens
- Estrogens
- Progestins
- Leuprolide
- Goserelin
- Narfarelin

- Tamoxifen
- Toremifene
- Flutamide
- Anastrozole
- Letrozole

Monoclonal antibodies
- Rituximab
- Trastuzumab

*Antitumor antibiotics are italicized; plant alkaloids are underlined.

PHASES OF THE CELL CYCLE

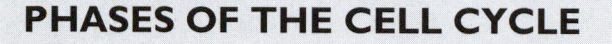

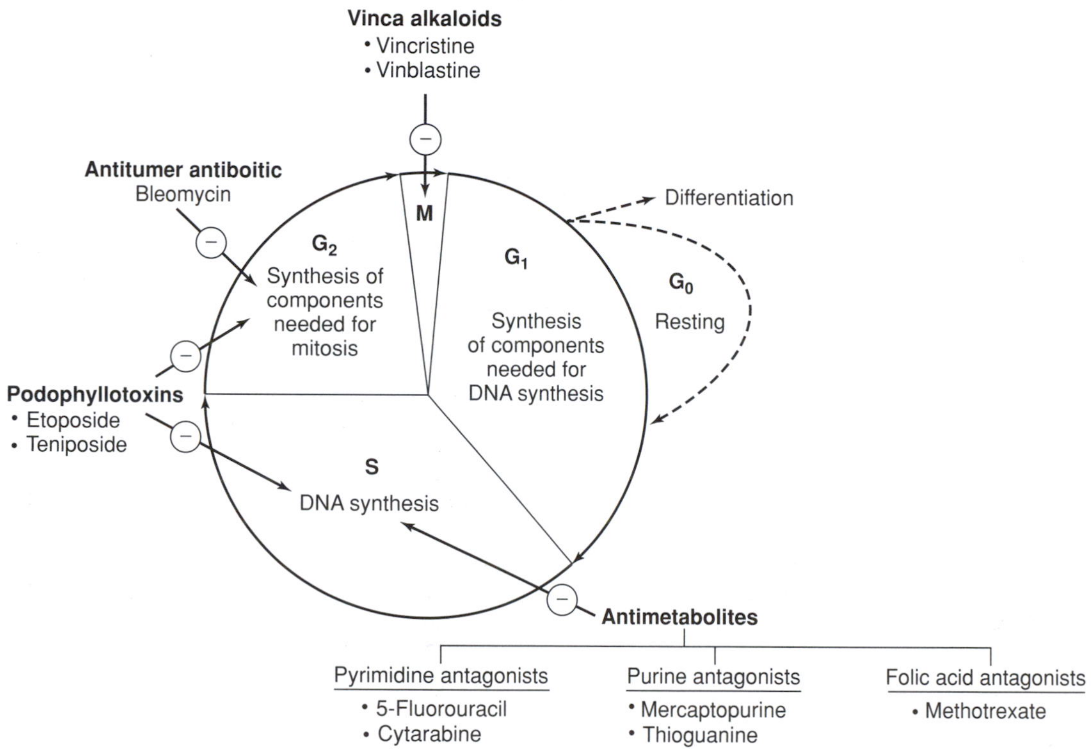

Vinca alkaloids
- Vincristine
- Vinblastine

Antitumer antiboitic
Bleomycin

Differentiation

M

G$_2$
Synthesis of components needed for mitosis

G$_1$
Synthesis of components needed for DNA synthesis

G$_0$
Resting

Podophyllotoxins
- Etoposide
- Teniposide

S
DNA synthesis

Antimetabolites

Pyrimidine antagonists	Purine antagonists	Folic acid antagonists
• 5-Fluorouracil	• Mercaptopurine	• Methotrexate
• Cytarabine	• Thioguanine	

All cells—normal and neoplastic—must traverse these cell cycle phases before and during cell division. CCS drug actions may not be restricted to a specific phase, but tumor cells are usually most responsive to specific drugs (or drug groups) in the phases indicated. Cell cycle-nonspecific (CCNS) drugs act on tumor cells while they are actively cycling and while they are in the resting phase (G$_0$).

Modified from Katzung BG, ed: *Basic & Clinical Pharmacology*, 8th ed, p 926. Originally published by Appleton & Lange. © 2001 by the McGraw-Hill Companies, Inc.

II. Alkylating Drugs

Mechanism of Action: Alkylating agents have a very reactive chemical moiety that binds to the bases of DNA causing damage that is very difficult to repair and sometimes irreparable.

Resistance Mechanisms: Four resistance mechanisms counteract the effects of alkylating agents:

1. Decreased transport in those that are actively transported into the cells
2. Increased pumping of the drug out of the cell
3. Increased ability to repair the DNA damage
4. Increased glutathione levels to get rid of the reactive species

ALKYLATING DRUG FACTS

Drug	Pharmacokinetics	Mechanism of Action	Clinical Uses and General Information	Side Effects
Mechlorethamine (Mustargen)	• **A:** IV or intracavitary • **M:** Undergoes rapid chemical transformation and combines with water or reactive compounds of cells	• Nitrogen mustard analogue • Interferes with DNA replication and transcription of RNA	• Lymphoma (Hodgkin's and non-Hodgkin's) • Malignant effusions • More stable and easier to use than nitrogen mustard	• Bone marrow suppression • Headache • Injection site reaction • Nausea • Vomiting • Weakness
Cyclophosphamide (Cytoxan)	• **A:** PO and IV • **M:** Undergoes hepatic activation to combine with water or reactive compounds of cells • **E:** Parent drug and metabolites excreted in urine	• Cross links RNA and DNA • Inhibits protein synthesis (by cross-linking DNA and RNA)	• Breast CA • Lymphoma (Hodgkin's and non-Hodgkin's) • Multiple myeloma • Neuroblastoma • Carcinomas • Longer acting and more stable analogues of nitrogen mustard	• Bone marrow suppression • Nausea • Vomiting • Hemorrhagic cystitis • Bladder fibrosis • Bladder carcinoma • Sterility • Alopecia

Continued

ALKYLATING DRUG FACTS (Continued)

Drug	Pharmacokinetics	Mechanism of Action	Clinical Uses and General Information	Side Effects
Ifosfamide (IFEX)			• Testicular germ cell tumors	• Encephalopathy • Hemorrhagic cystitis • Leukopenia • Thrombocytopenia
Chlorambucil (Leukeran)	• **A:** PO • **M:** Hepatic metabolism • **E:** Parent drug and metabolites excreted in urine	• Cross links DNA strands	• Chronic lymphocytic leukemia • Lymphoma (Hodgkin's and non-Hodgkin's)	• Allergic reactions (urticaria to hypersensitivity) • Bone marrow suppression • GI distress
Melphalan (Alkeran)	• **A:** PO and IV • **M:** Spontaneous hydrolysis in plasma • **E:** Majority of parent drug and metabolites excreted in urine; remainder in feces		• Melanoma • Multiple myeloma • Ovarian CA	
Busulfan (Myleran, Busulfex)	• **A:** PO and IV • **M:** Hepatic metabolism • **E:** Metabolites excreted in urine		• Chronic myelogenous leukemia • Myeloablation prior to stem cell transplant	• Allergic reactions • Bone marrow suppression • GI distress • Pulmonary fibrosis • Hyperpigmentation
Lomustine (CeeNU)	• **A:** PO • **M:** Hepatic metabolism • **E:** Majority of metabolites excreted in urine	• Inhibits DNA synthesis • Interferes with the action of DNA and RNA	• Brain tumors • Hodgkin's lymphoma	• Bone marrow suppression • GI distress • Hepatotoxicity • Pulmonary fibrosis • Neurotoxicity

Drug	Pharmacokinetics	Mechanism of Action	Indications	Toxicity
Carmustine (BiCNU, Gliadel)	• **A:** IV and intracranial wafer • **M:** Hepatic metabolism • **E:** Majority of metabolites excreted in urine	• Inhibition of DNA and RNA synthesis	• Brain tumors • Lymphoma (Hodgkin's and non-Hodgkin's) • Melanoma • Multiple myeloma	• Bone marrow suppression • GI distress • Hepatotoxicity • Pulmonary fibrosis
Streptozocin (Zanosar)	• **A:** IV • **M:** Hepatic metabolism • **E:** Majority of metabolites excreted in urine	• Inhibition of DNA synthesis	• Pancreatic CA	• Nephrotoxicity • Neurotoxicity
Cisplatin (Platinol)	• **A:** IV • **M:** Nonenzymatic conversion to inactive metabolites • **E:** Majority of metabolites excreted in urine	• Exact MOA unknown • May cross link DNA	• Bladder CA • Ovarian CA • Testicular CA	• Bone marrow suppression • GI distress • Hepatotoxicity • Nephrotoxicity • Neurotoxicity • Ototoxicity
Carboplatin (Paraplatin)	• **A:** IV • **M:** Hydrolysis in plasma to active metabolite • **E:** Metabolites excreted in urine		• Ovarian CA	• Bone marrow suppression • GI distress • Neurotoxicity • Ototoxicity
Dacarbazine (Dtic-Dome)	• **A:** IV • **M:** Hepatic metabolism • **E:** Parent drug and metabolites excreted in urine	• Exact MOA unknown • May inhibit DNA and RNA synthesis via formation of carbonium ions	• Malignant melanoma • Hodgkin's lymphoma	• Bone marrow suppression • Hepatotoxicity • GI distress

Continued

ALKYLATING DRUG FACTS (Continued)

Drug	Pharmacokinetics	Mechanism of Action	Clinical Uses and General Information	Side Effects
Procarbazine (Matulane, Natulan)	• **A:** PO • **M:** Hepatic metabolism • **E:** Majority of metabolites excreted in urine	• Exact MOA unknown • May inhibit DNA, RNA, and protein synthesis	• Brain tumors • Hodgkin's lymphoma	• Bone marrow suppression • GI distress • Hepatotoxicity • Neurotoxicity
Altretamine/ Hexamethylmelamine (Hexalen)	• **A:** PO • **M:** Hepatic metabolism by P450 enzymes • **E:** Metabolites excreted in urine		• Ovarian CA	• GI distress • Hepatotoxicity • Neurotoxicity

III. Antimetabolites

Pharmacokinetics: Because nucleoside triphosphates, the building blocks of DNA, are too polar to enter the cell, all of these drugs must be taken into the cell as a prodrug and then activated.

Mechanism of Action: All of the antimetabolites are structural analogues of the normal building blocks of DNA. They either are incorrectly incorporated into the DNA—which halts its production—or they inhibit the enzymes involved in the synthesis of DNA building blocks. These only work during the S phase of the cell cycle.

ANTIMETABOLITES: PYRIMIDINE, PURINE, AND FOLIC ACID ANTAGONISTS

Drug	Pharmacokinetics	Mechanisms of Action and Resistance	Clinical Uses	Side Effects
Pyrimidine Antagonists				
5-Fluorouracil/ 5-FU (Adrucil)	• **A:** IV • **M:** Metabolized in liver and tissues • **E:** Metabolites are exhaled and excreted in urine	• Active metabolite inhibits thymidylate synthase • Results in decreased DNA synthesis • Decreased activation of 5-FU • Increased thymidylate synthase activity • Reduced drug sensitivity of that enzyme	• Bladder CA • Breast CA • GI CAs • Head and neck CA • Liver CA • Ovarian CA	• Alopecia • GI distress • White blood cell dysfunction • Photosensitivity
Cytosine arabinoside/ Ara-C/ Cytarabine (Cytosar-U)	• **A:** IV, SC, or intrathecal • **M:** Metabolized in liver, kidneys, GI mucosa, granulocytes • **E:** Metabolites excreted in urine	• Active metabolite inhibits DNA polymerase • Decreased conversion to active metabolite • Decreased uptake of the drug	• Acute leukemias	• GI distress • Myelosuppression • Neurotoxicity

Continued

ANTIMETABOLITES: PYRIMIDINE, PURINE, AND FOLIC ACID ANTAGONISTS (Continued)

Drug	Pharmacokinetics	Mechanisms of Action and Resistance	Clinical Uses	Side Effects
Purine Antagonists				
Mercaptopurine/ 6-MP (Purinethol)	• **A:** PO • **M:** Hepatic metabolism • **E:** Parent drug and metabolites excreted in urine	• Active metabolites decrease de novo purine synthesis and cause DNA strand breaks • Decreased activity of the enzyme that activates these drugs • Increased production of alkaline phosphatases that inactivate the toxic metabolites	• Leukemias • Lymphomas (not chronic lymphocytic leukemia or Hodgkin's)	• GI distress • Hepatotoxicity • Bone marrow suppression
Thioguanine/ 6-TG (Tabloid)				
Folic Acid Antagonist				
Methotrexate/ MTX (Folex, Abitrexate)	• **A:** PO, IV, IM, and intrathecal • **E:** Majority excreted unchanged in urine	• Substrate for an inhibitor of dihydrofolate reductase, an enzyme in the pathway of purine synthesis • Decreased drug accumulation • Change in dihydrofolate reductase	• Breast CA • Head and neck CA • Non–small cell and small cell lung CA • Gestational trophoblastic neoplasms • Leukemias • Lymphomas • Choriocarcinoma • Sarcomas • Abortion • Ectopic pregnancy • RA • Psoriasis	• GI distress • Hepatotoxicity • Bone marrow suppression • Nephrotoxicity

IV. Antitumor Antibiotics

ACTION OF ANTITUMOR ANTIBIOTICS

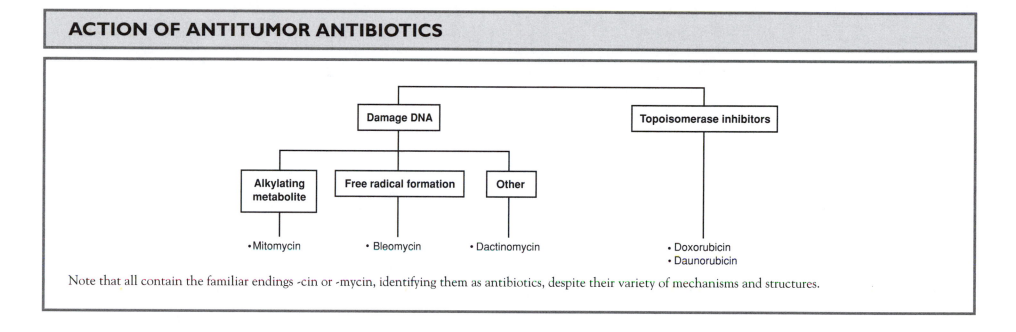

Note that all contain the familiar endings -cin or -mycin, identifying them as antibiotics, despite their variety of mechanisms and structures.

ANTITUMOR ANTIBIOTICS: CELL CYCLE-SPECIFIC AND CELL CYCLE-NONSPECIFIC DRUGS

Drug	Pharmacokinetics	Mechanism of Action	Clinical Uses	Side Effects
Cell Cyclic-Specific				
Bleomycin (Blenoxane)	• **A:** IV • **M:** Metabolized in tissues throughout the body • **E:** Majority excreted unchanged in urine	• Generates free radicals that bind to DNA • Causes DNA strand breaks in both single and double strands • Act ONLY during the G2 phase of the cell cycle	• Head and neck CA • Cervical CA • Testicular CA • Lymphoma	• Hypersensitivity reactions • Pulmonary toxicity • Mucocutaneous reactions (alopecia, hyperkeratosis)
Cell Cycle-Nonspecific				
Doxorubicin (Adriamycin)	• **A:** IV • **M:** Hepatic metabolism • **E:** Majority of parent drug and metabolites excreted in feces; remainder in urine	• Inhibit topoisomerase II • Induce cells to undergo apoptosis • Generate free radicals	• Bladder CA • Breast CA • Gastric CA • Leukemia • Neuroblastoma • Ovarian CA • Small cell lung CA • Thyroid CA • Myeloma • Sarcomas • Hodgkin's lymphoma	• Cardiotoxicity (conductive toxicities and CHF) • Facial flushing • Necrotizing colitis • Red discoloration of urine • Alopecia
Daunorubicin (Cerubidine)			• Leukemia	

Mitomycin (Mutamycin) *[handwritten: ADR all organs, tx CAs]*	• **A:** IV • **M:** Metabolized at multiple sites, including the liver • **E:** Majority of parent drug and metabolites excreted in urine; remainder in feces	• Metabolized by liver enzymes to form an alkylating agent that cross links DNA	• Adenocarcinomas of the stomach and pancreas • Breast CA • Cervical CA • Non–small cell lung CA • Stomach CA	• Cardiotoxicity • Hepatotoxicity • Nephrotoxicity • Myelosuppression • Pulmonary toxicity
Dactinomycin (Cosmegen)	• **A:** IV • **E:** Parent drug and metabolites excreted in urine and feces	• Binds to ds-DNA and inhibits DNA dependent RNA synthesis, causing strand breaks	• Ewing's sarcoma • Rhabdomyosarcoma • Testicular CA • Trophoblastic neoplasms • Wilms' tumor	• Bone marrow suppression • Skin reactions • GI irritation

V. Plant Alkaloids

PLANT ALKALOIDS BY ACTION AND CLASS

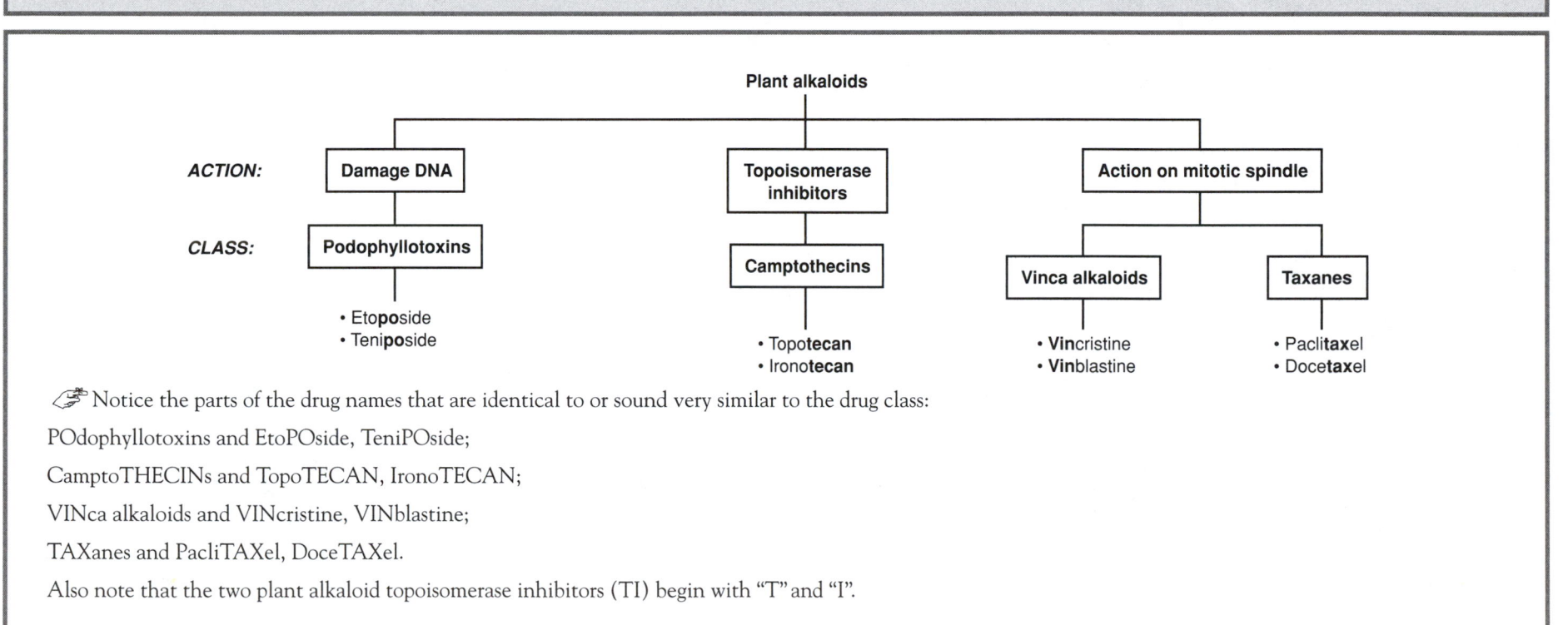

☞ Notice the parts of the drug names that are identical to or sound very similar to the drug class:

POdophyllotoxins and EtoPOside, TeniPOside;

CamptoTHECINs and TopoTECAN, IronoTECAN;

VINca alkaloids and VINcristine, VINblastine;

TAXanes and PacliTAXel, DoceTAXel.

Also note that the two plant alkaloid topoisomerase inhibitors (TI) begin with "T" and "I".

PLANT ALKALOIDS: DRUG FACTS

Drug	Pharmacokinetics	Mechanism of Action	Clinical Uses	Side Effects
Vinca Alkaloids				
Vincristine (Vincasar, Oncovin)	• **A:** IV • **M:** Hepatic metabolism by P450 enzymes • **E:** Metabolites excreted in feces and urine	• Spindle poisons that bind to the tubulin necessary for midline alignment of chromosomes and separation to the poles in mitosis • Increase apoptosis signals • Most effective during the M phase of the cell cycle	• AIDS-related Kaposi's sarcoma • Leukemia • Lymphoma • Neuroblastoma • Rhabdomyosarcoma • Small cell lung CA	• Constipation • Dysuria • Neurotoxic actions • Paralytic ileus
Vinblastine (Velban, Velsar)			• AIDS-related Kaposi's sarcoma • Bladder CA • Leukemia • Lymphoma • Small cell lung CA • Testicular CA	• Alopecia • Constipation • Leukopenia • Malaise • Pain at tumor site • Bone marrow suppression
Podophyllotoxins				
Etoposide (VP-16, VePesid)	• **A:** IV • **M:** Hepatic metabolism • **E:** Majority of parent drug and metabolites excreted in urine; remainder in feces	• Increases degradation of DNA • Inhibits mitochondrial electron transport • Topoisomerase inhibitors • Most effective during late S and early G2 phases of the cell cycle	• Leukemias • Lung CA • Ovarian CA • Testicular CA • Neuroblastoma • Prostate CA	• Alopecia • Leukopenia • GI distress • Thrombocytopenia

Continued

PLANT ALKALOIDS: DRUG FACTS (Continued)

Drug	Pharmacokinetics	Mechanism of Action	Clinical Uses	Side Effects
Teniposide (Vumon)	• A: IV • E: Majority excreted unchanged in urine; remainder in feces		• Leukemia	
Camptothecins				
Topotecan (Hycamtin)	• A: IV • M: pH-dependent hydrolysis; minor hepatic metabolism • E: Majority of parent drug and metabolites excreted in urine; remainder in feces	• Inhibit topoisomerase I • Results in DNA damage	• Ovarian CA • Small cell lung CA	• Alopecia • Anemia • GI distress • Neutropenia • Thrombocytopenia
Irinotecan (Camptosar)	• A: IV • M: Prodrug metabolized to active metabolite in the liver • E: Parent drug and metabolites excreted in urine and feces		• Colon CA • Rectal CA	• GI distress (especially severe diarrhea) • Leukopenia • Neutropenia

Taxanes				
Paclitaxel (Taxol)	• **A:** IV • **M:** Hepatic metabolism by P450 enzymes • **E:** Majority of parent drug and metabolites excreted in feces; remainder in urine	• **Spindle poisons** that prevent microtubule disassembly into tubulin monomers • **Disrupt mitosis**	• Advanced breast CA • Bladder CA • Cervical CA • Esophageal CA • Head and neck CA • Ovarian CAs • Non–small cell lung CA • Small cell lung CA	• Hypersensitivity reactions during infusion • Peripheral neuropathy • Neutropenia • Thrombocytopenia
Docetaxel (Taxotere)			• Breast CA • Non–small cell lung CA	• Anemia • Cardiovascular side effects • Neurotoxicity • Neutropenia • Thrombocytopenia

VI. Hormonal Anticancer Drugs

CLASSIFICATION OF HORMONAL ANTICANCER DRUGS

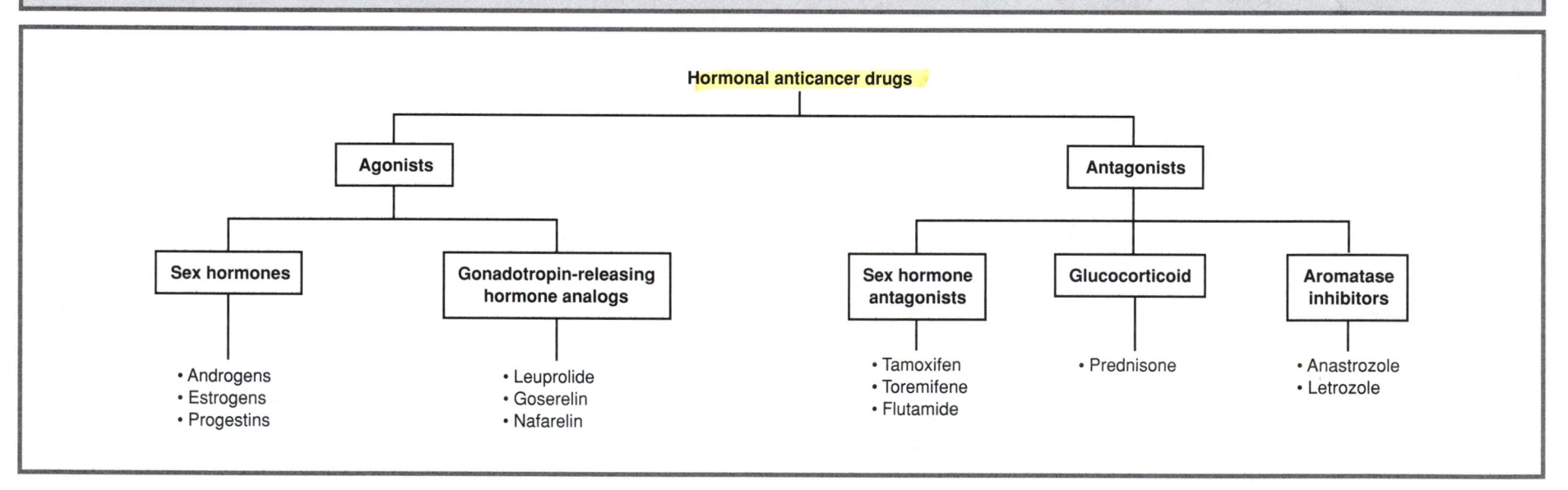

HORMONAL ANTICANCER DRUG FACTS

Drug/Group	Route of Administration	Mechanism of Action	Clinical Uses	Side Effects
Glucocorticoids				
Prednisone (Deltasone)	• PO	• Anti-inflammatory via inhibition of the inflammatory cells • Exact mechanism unknown • May trigger apoptosis	• Acute and chronic lymphocytic leukemia • Hodgkin's lymphoma • Non-Hodgkin's lymphoma	• Adrenal suppression • Osteoporosis • Redistribution of body fat • Cushing-like symptoms • Cataracts • Hypertension ↑ glucose • Ulcers • Acne
Sex Hormones				
Androgens Estrogens Progestins	• Refer to Chapter 9: VI. Drugs Affecting Reproductive Hormones	• Alter hormone balance to not favor tumor growth	• Androgens tend to be used in breast CAs • Estrogens are used in prostate CA	• Varies with hormone
Sex Hormone Antagonists				
Tamoxifen (Nolvadex)	• PO	• Estrogen-receptor partial agonist/antagonist	• Receptor-positive breast CA	• GI distress (nausea and vomiting) • Hot flashes • Hypercalcemia • Ocular dysfunction • Peripheral edema • Vaginal bleeding

Continued

HORMONAL ANTICANCER DRUG FACTS (Continued)

Drug/Group	Route of Administration	Mechanism of Action	Clinical Uses	Side Effects
Toremifene (Fareston)		• Estrogen-receptor antagonist	• Breast CA	• Hepatotoxicity • Hot flashes • Nausea
Flutamide (Eulexin)		• Androgen-receptor antagonist	• Prostate CA	• Gynecomastia • Hot flashes • Hepatic dysfunction
Gonadotropin-Releasing Hormone Analogs				
Leuprolide (Lupron)	• SC, IM, implant	• GnRH agonists • Inhibit release of pituitary luteinizing hormone and follicle-stimulating hormone	• Prostate CA	• Bone pain (leuprolide) • Gynecomastia • Hematuria • Impotence • Testicular atrophy
Goserelin (Zoladex)	• SC			
Nafarelin (Synarel)	• Nasal spray			
Aromatase Inhibitors				
Anastrozole (Arimidex)	• PO	• Inhibit aromatase, the enzyme that catalyzes the conversion of androstenedione to estrone	• Advanced breast CA	• Bone and back pain • Dyspnea • GI distress (nausea and diarrhea) • Hot flashes
Letrozole (Femara)				

VII. Chemotherapeutic Drugs

MISCELLANEOUS CHEMOTHERAPEUTICS: DRUG FACTS

Drug	Pharmacokinetics	Mechanism of Action	Clinical Uses	Side Effects
Amsacrine (AMSA)	• **A:** IV • **M:** Hepatic metabolism • **E:** Metabolites excreted in urine and feces	• Intercalates into DNA by binding to A-T pairs causing DNA strand breaks	• Acute leukemia	• Anemia • GI distress • Leukopenia • Thrombocytopenia
Asparaginase (Elspar)	• **A:** IV and IM • **M:** Metabolic fate unknown • **E:** Only trace amounts recovered in urine	• An enzyme that degrades asparagine, an essential amino acid for tumor cell growth	• Acute leukemia	• Bleeding • Hypersensitivity reactions • Pancreatitis
Mitoxantrone (Novantrone)	• **A:** IV • **M:** Hepatic metabolism • **E:** Metabolites excreted in urine and feces	• Exact mechanism of action unknown • Might act via alkylation of DNA bases	• Acute leukemia • Prostate CA • Relapsing multiple sclerosis	• Cough/shortness of breath • GI distress • Leukopenia • Thrombocytopenia • Renal failure

CHEMOTHERAPEUTICS: MONOCLONAL ANTIBODIES

Drug	Route of Administration	Mechanism of Action	Clinical Uses	Side Effects
Rituximab (Rituxan)	• IV	• A mouse/human chimera • Monoclonal antibody that has anti-CD20+ properties that then attacks normal and malignant B cells, which also possess CD20+	• Hodgkin's lymphoma	• Allergic reaction • Cardiotoxicity (CHF) • Infusion reaction
Trastuzumab (Herceptin)		• Monoclonal Ab against HER2 protein, a surface protein over expressed in breast cancer	• Breast CA	• Chill • Fever • Headache • Nausea • Vomiting

CHAPTER 11
IMMUNOMODULATORS

TERMS TO LEARN

Aplastic Anemia	Low blood count due to defective regeneration of cells.
Erythema Nodosum Leprosum	Painful erythematous subcutaneous nodules seen in patients with a high level of mycobacterial antigens.
Hirsutism	Excessive body and facial hair in women.
Kawasaki Disease	Medium to large vessel vasculitis seen in children; symptoms include conjunctivitis, rash, erythema of the palms and soles, coronary aneurysms, and strawberry tongue.
Malignant Osteopetrosis	Increased skeletal density due to osteoclastic failure.

I. Drugs that Influence the Immune Response

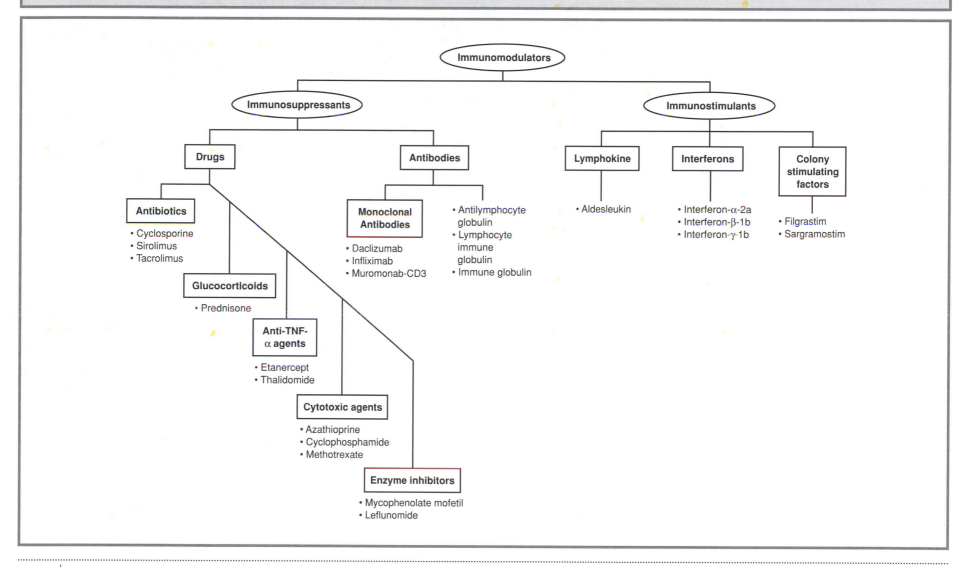

Immunomodulators

- Immunosuppressants
  - Drugs
    - Antibiotics
      - Cyclosporine
      - Sirolimus
      - Tacrolimus
    - Glucocorticoids
      - Prednisone
    - Anti-TNF-α agents
      - Etanercept
      - Thalidomide
    - Cytotoxic agents
      - Azathioprine
      - Cyclophosphamide
      - Methotrexate
    - Enzyme inhibitors
      - Mycophenolate mofetil
      - Leflunomide
  - Antibodies
    - Monoclonal Antibodies
      - Daclizumab
      - Infliximab
      - Muromonab-CD3
    - Antilymphocyte globulin
    - Lymphocyte immune globulin
    - Immune globulin
- Immunostimulants
  - Lymphokine
    - Aldesleukin
  - Interferons
    - Interferon-α-2a
    - Interferon-β-1b
    - Interferon-γ-1b
  - Colony stimulating factors
    - Filgrastim
    - Sargramostim

II. Immunosuppressants

IMMUNOSUPPRESSANTS: DRUG FACTS

Drug	Pharmacokinetics	Mechanism of Action	Clinical Uses	Side Effects
Fungal Cyclic Peptide Antibiotic				
Cyclosporine (Neoral)	• **A:** PO or IV • **M:** Metabolized by hepatic P450 enzymes • **E:** Metabolites excreted in feces	• Binds to cyclophilin to form a complex that inhibits calcineurin • Highly selective inhibition of T cell activation by blocking cytokine production (especially IL-2)	• Prophylaxis for organ rejection following transplant (ie, kidney, heart, liver, BMT, lung, and pancreas) • Treatment of graft versus host reactions (often in combination with corticosteroids) • Autoimmune disorders (ie, RA and severe psoriasis)	• Gingival hyperplasia • GI distress • Hirsutism • Hypertension • Nephrotoxicity • Neurologic effects (seizures and tremor)
Macrolide Antibiotics				
Sirolimus / Rapamycin (Rapamune)	• **A:** PO • **M:** Metabolized by hepatic P450 enzymes • **E:** Metabolites excreted in feces	• Binds to FK-binding protein, inhibiting the response of T cells to cytokines without affecting cytokine production	• Liver and kidney transplantation • Potentially useful in conjunction with cyclosporine with which it acts synergistically	• Blood dyscrasias • Hyperlipidemia • Hypertension • Rash
Tacrolimus / FK-506 (Prograf)	• **A:** PO or IV • **M:** Metabolized by hepatic P450 enzymes • **E:** Metabolites excreted in feces	• Binds to FK-binding protein and forms a complex that inhibits calcineurin • Calcineurin regulates the T cells ability to produce interleukins	• 10–100 times more potent immunosuppression than cyclosporine • Liver and kidney transplantation	• Asthenia • Blood dyscrasias • GI distress • Hyperglycemia • Nephrotoxicity • Neurotoxicity

Glucocorticoid

| Prednisone | • **A:** PO
• **M:** Metabolized in liver and other tissues to active metabolite, prednisolone
• **E:** Metabolites excreted in urine | • Impaired release of cytokines from macrophages and granulocytes
• Suppression of T cell proliferation and activation
• Suppression of antibody production
• Reduction of accumulation of macrophages
• Seems to spare B cell population under normal conditions
• Inhibit migration of cells that cause acute rejection of an organ, which is an inflammatory response | • Administered before, during, and after transplant surgery (always used in combination with other immunosuppressants, such as cyclosporine, for organ transplantation
• Autoimmune diseases (eg, RA, SLE, and hemolytic anemia)
• Treatment of acute graft versus host rejection (suppress secondary [antibody] response via B cell suppression)
• Attenuation of allergic reactions | • Adrenal suppression (cushingoid reactions) associated with an inability to regulate endogenous glucocorticoid levels following use
• Osteoporosis (LTU)
• Redistribution of body fat
• Inhibition of growth |

Anti TNF-α Agents

| Etanercept (Enbrel) | • **A:** SC
• **M:** Possibly metabolized by reticuloendothelial system | • Solution of TNF receptor
• Acts as a competitive inhibitor of TNF | • Treatment of RA and juvenile RA | • Aplastic anemia
• CNS symptoms suggestive of demyelinating conditions
• Hypertension or hypotension
• Infections |

Continued

IMMUNOSUPPRESSANTS: DRUG FACTS (Continued)

Drug	Pharmacokinetics	Mechanism of Action	Clinical Uses	Side Effects
Thalidomide (Thalomid)	• **A:** PO • **M:** Undergoes nonenzymatic hydrolysis, also seems to be metabolized by hepatic P450 enzymes • **E:** Metabolites excreted in urine	• May act as a selective inhibitor of TNF-α	• Treatment and prophylaxis of erythema nodosum leprosum	• Dizziness • Drowsiness • GI distress (diarrhea, nausea, constipation, abdominal pain) • Peripheral neuropathy
Cytotoxic Agents				
Azathioprine (Imuran)	• **A:** PO and IV • **M:** Prodrug slowly converted in tissues to the antimetabolite mercaptopurine • **E:** Metabolites excreted in feces	• Blocks de novo purine synthesis and interferes with DNA synthesis • Somewhat more effect on T cells than B cells	• Autoimmune diseases (ie, RA, SLE) • Prophylaxis of rejection in renal transplants	• Bone marrow suppression • Rash • GI disturbances • Some hepatotoxicity
Cyclophosphamide (Cytoxan)	• **A:** PO, IV, IM, and intracavitary • **M:** Hepatic metabolism • **E:** Parent drug and metabolites excreted in urine	• Inhibits DNA and RNA synthesis via cross-linking of these molecules • Destroys any proliferating lymphoid cells (more effective suppression of B cell proliferation)	• Autoimmune diseases (eg, multiple sclerosis, SLE, and RA) • Chemotherapy	• Amenorrhea • Severe nausea and vomiting • Hemorrhagic cystitis • Cardiotoxic
Methotrexate / MTX (Trexall)	• **A:** PO, IM, IV, and intrathecal • **E:** Majority excreted unchanged in urine	• Inhibits dihydrofolate reductase blocking synthesis of nucleoside phosphates inhibiting DNA synthesis • Rapidly proliferating cells are destroyed	• Treatment of autoimmune diseases (eg, RA and psoriasis) • Chemotherapy • Combined therapy with cyclosporine with graft versus host reactions following BMT	• GI tract irritation • Hepatotoxicity • Thrombocytopenia

Enzyme Inhibitors

Mycophenolate Mofetil (Cellcept)	• **A:** PO and IV • **M:** Metabolized presystemically to active metabolite • **E:** Metabolites excreted primarily in urine	• Metabolite (MPA) inhibits inosine monophosphate dehydrogenase, an enzyme in the de novo purine synthesis pathway • Blocks de novo purine synthesis • Results in inhibition of B and T lymphocyte proliferation	• Prophylaxis for heart, liver, and kidney transplant rejection • Typically used with cyclosporine and prednisone	• Few GI disturbances
Leflunomide (Arava)	• **A:** PO • **M:** Believed to be metabolized in GI wall and liver • **E:** Metabolites excreted in urine and feces	• Inhibits dihydroorotate dehydrogenase, an enzyme in the de novo pyrimidine synthesis pathway • Blocks de novo pyrimidine synthesis • Results in inhibition of B and T lymphocyte proliferation	• Treatment of RA	• Alopecia • GI distress (diarrhea, nausea, constipation, abdominal pain) • Hepatotoxicity • Hypertension • URI • UTI

ANTIBODY IMMUNOSUPPRESSANT FACTS

Drug	Mechanism of Action	Clinical Uses	Side Effects
All of these antibody immunosuppressants are administered intravenously.			
Antilymphocyte Globulin / Lymphocyte Immune Globulin (Atgam)	• Antibodies that bind to T lymphocytes causing them to be destroyed by complement	• Treatment of acute rejection following kidney transplants • Prophylaxis for rejection following kidney transplants • Treatment of aplastic anemia in patients not suitable for BMT • Prophylaxis for acute graft versus host disease following BMT	• Hypersensitivity reactions (anaphylaxis, serum sickness)
Immune Globulin Intravenous / IGIV / IVIG	• Precise mechanism of action unknown • May act via increase of suppressor T cells or diminution of helper T cells	• Treatment of patients with immunodeficiency syndromes • Treatment of Kawasaki syndrome (reduction of systemic inflammation and prevention of coronary aneurysms) • Treatment of severe asthma • Treatment of some autoimmune diseases (eg, idiopathic thrombocytopenic purpura, multiple sclerosis, and SLE)	• Dyspnea • Hypersensitivity reactions • Tachycardia
Daclizumab (Zenapax)	• Binds to the α subunit of the IL-2 receptor on T cells, preventing activation by IL-2	• Prophylaxis for rejection following kidney transplants	• Chest pain • Dyspnea • Fever • GI distress (nausea, vomiting) • Hypotension or hypertension

Infliximab (Remicade)	• Antibody targeted against TNF-α (mediates inflammation and modulates cellular immune response)	• Treatment of autoimmune disease (eg, RA, psoriatic arthritis) • Treatment of Crohn's disease	• GI distress (abdominal pain, nausea, vomiting) • Infusion related reactions (fevers, chills, pruritus, chest pain, dyspnea, hypotension, myalgia)
Muromonab-CD3 (Orthoclone OKT3)	• Directed towards CD3 molecule on the surface of all T cells • Causes initial release of cytokines • Eventually results in inhibition of T cells	• Treatment of acute rejection following kidney, heart, or liver transplants	• Blood dyscrasias • Cytokine release syndrome (flu-like symptoms) • Hearing loss • Hypersensitivity reactions • Impaired vision • Neurologic reactions (headache, seizures)

SITES OF ACTION OF IMMUNOSUPPRESSIVE DRUGS

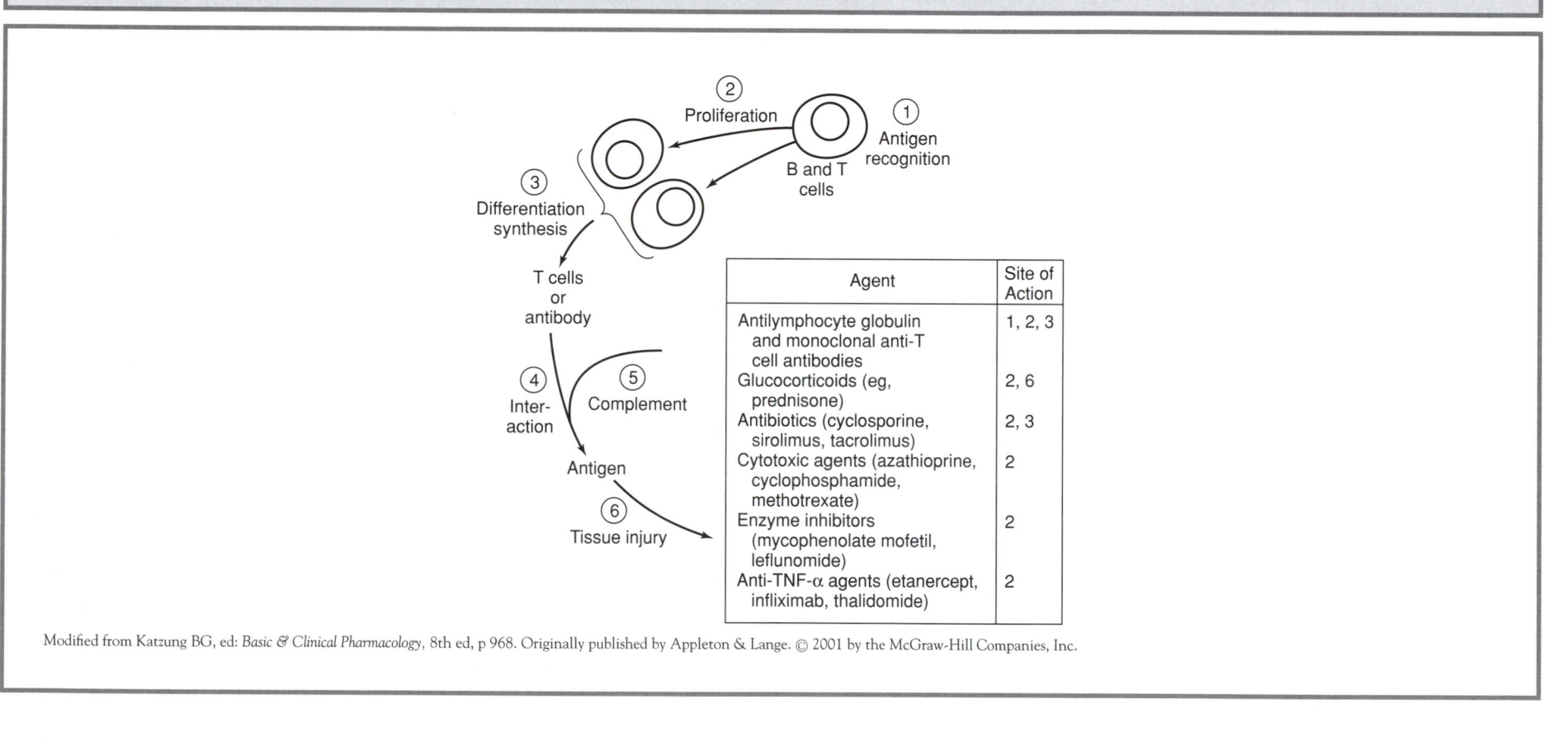

Agent	Site of Action
Antilymphocyte globulin and monoclonal anti-T cell antibodies	1, 2, 3
Glucocorticoids (eg, prednisone)	2, 6
Antibiotics (cyclosporine, sirolimus, tacrolimus)	2, 3
Cytotoxic agents (azathioprine, cyclophosphamide, methotrexate)	2
Enzyme inhibitors (mycophenolate mofetil, leflunomide)	2
Anti-TNF-α agents (etanercept, infliximab, thalidomide)	2

Modified from Katzung BG, ed: *Basic & Clinical Pharmacology*, 8th ed, p 968. Originally published by Appleton & Lange. © 2001 by the McGraw-Hill Companies, Inc.

III. Immunostimulants

IMMUNOSTIMULANTS: DRUG FACTS

Drug	Class	Administration	Mechanism of Action	Clinical Uses	Side Effects
Aldesleukin (Proleukin)	• IL-2 lymphokine	• IV	• Increases lymphokine-activated killer cells and helper T cells	• Malignant melanoma • Renal cell carcinoma	• Blood dyscrasias • GI distress (nausea, vomiting, diarrhea) • Hepatotoxicity • Hypotension • Nephrotoxicity • Pulmonary toxicity
Interferon-α-2a (Roferon, Intron)	• Interferons • Glycoproteins	• SC	• Enhance Ag presentation • Enhance activation of natural killer cells, macrophages, and cytotoxic T cells	• Chronic hepatitis C • Chronic myelogenous leukemia • Hairy cell leukemia • Kaposi's sarcoma	• Depression • GI distress (nausea, vomiting, diarrhea, anorexia, abdominal pain) • Flu-like symptoms (fatigue, myalgia, fever, chills) • Injection site reaction
Interferon-β-1b (Betaseron)				• Relapsing-remitting multiple sclerosis	• Flu-like symptoms (fatigue, myalgia, fever, chills) • Injection site reaction

Continued

IMMUNOSTIMULANTS: DRUG FACTS (Continued)

Drug	Class	Administration	Mechanism of Action	Clinical Uses	Side Effects
Interferon-γ-1b (Actimmune)			• Enhance Ag presentation • Enhance activation of natural killer cells, macrophages, and cytotoxic T cells • Also seems to increase synthesis of TNF	• Chronic granulomatous disease • Malignant osteopetrosis	• GI distress (nausea, vomiting, diarrhea, anorexia, abdominal pain) • Flu-like symptoms (fatigue, myalgia, fever, chills) • Injection site reaction
Filgrastim (Neupogen)	• Colony stimulating factor	• IV and SC	• Induce proliferation and maturation of various myeloid cells	• Severe chronic neutropenia • BMT recipients • Treatment of cancer patients receiving myelosuppressive chemotherapy	• Skeletal pain
Sargramostim (Leukine)		• IV		• Following induction chemotherapy in acute myelogenous leukemia • Myeloid reconstitution after allogenic BMT	• Arthralgia • Headache • Myalgia • Pericardial effusion

DRUGS USED TO TREAT INFLAMMATION

TERMS TO LEARN

Abortifacient	An agent that causes an abortion.
Dysmenorrhea	Painful menstruation.
Orthostatic Hypotension	Low blood pressure in the standing position.
Tinnitis	Ringing in the ears.

I. Prostaglandin Analogs

PROSTAGLANDIN ANALOGS: DRUG FACTS

Drug	Pharmacokinetics	Clinical Uses	Side Effects
PGE₁ Analog			
Alprostadil (Prostin, Muse, Caverject)	• **A:** IV, intracavernosal injection, and intraurethral suppository • **M:** Metabolized in the lungs • **E:** Metabolites excreted in urine	• Maintains patent ductus arteriosus in infants with this condition or with congenital heart defects until surgical repair (Prostin) • Erectile dysfunction (Caverject, penile injection; Muse, suppository)	• Flushing • Bradycardia/tachycardia • Hypotension • Diarrhea • May result in gastric obstruction secondary to antral hyperplasia in neonates
Misoprostol (Cytotec)	• **A:** PO • **M:** Extensive first-pass metabolism (probably in GI tract) • **E:** Majority of metabolites excreted in urine; remainder in feces	• Treatment and prophylaxis of NSAID-induced gastric ulcer • Abortifacient • Cervical ripening and induction of labor	• GI effects (abdominal pain, diarrhea, constipation, and dyspepsia) • Headache • Vaginal bleeding

Continued

PROSTAGLANDIN ANALOGS: DRUG FACTS (Continued)

Drug	Pharmacokinetics	Clinical Uses	Side Effects
PGE₂ Analog Dinoprostone (Prepidil, ProstinE2, Cervidil)	• **A:** Vaginal gel and suppository • **M:** Metabolized in lungs, kidneys, spleen, and other tissues • **E:** Majority of parent drug and metabolites excreted in urine; remainder in feces	• Vaginal suppository to ripen cervix and induce labor (Prepidil - gel) • Induce abortion (Prostin E2 - vaginal suppository) • Both indications (Cervidil)	• Chills/shivering • GI effects (abdominal pain, diarrhea, nausea and vomiting) • Headache
PGI₂ Analog Epoprostenol (Flolan)	• **A:** IV • **M:** Hydrolyzed in plasma • **E:** Majority of metabolites excreted in urine; remainder in feces	• Pulmonary hypertension (drug of last resort, not very effective)	• Flushing • GI effects (abdominal pain, diarrhea, nausea and vomiting) • Headache • Hypotension

II. Drugs Used in the Treatment of Gout

MANAGING GOUT: DRUG FACTS				
Drug	**Pharmacokinetics**	**Mechanism of Action**	**Clinical Uses**	**Drawbacks and Side Effects**
Indomethacin (Indocin)	• **A:** PO, IV, or rectal • **M:** Hepatic metabolism • **E:** Parent drug and metabolites excreted in urine	• NSAID that inhibits COX • Reduces production of prostaglandins • Inhibits phagocytosis of uric acid crystal by macrophages	• Acute treatment of gouty arthritis	• GI effects (irritation, bleeding, and ulceration) • Renal effects (dysuria, interstitial nephritis, and renal failure) • CNS effects (headache, dizziness) • Hepatic effects (jaundice, cholestatic hepatitis) • Hematologic effects (thrombocytopenia, leukopenia)
Colchicine (Colsalide)	• **A:** PO and IV • **M:** Metabolized by the liver and other tissues • **E:** Metabolites excreted in feces and urine	• Disrupts the inflammatory cycle, which inhibits leukocyte migration and phagocytosis of uric acid crystals	• Acute treatment of gouty arthritis • Low doses useful for chronic treatment of gout	• Narrow therapeutic window so must be carefully titrated to effective dose in each individual • Overdose can lead to nephrotoxicity, hepatotoxicity, or death • Long $t_{1/2}$ in the white blood cells leading to systemic accumulation (must wait 3–4 days between uses) • IV dose must be administered in an indwelling catheter due to irritation • GI side effects (nausea, abdominal discomfort, vomiting, and diarrhea)

Continued

MANAGING GOUT: DRUG FACTS (Continued)

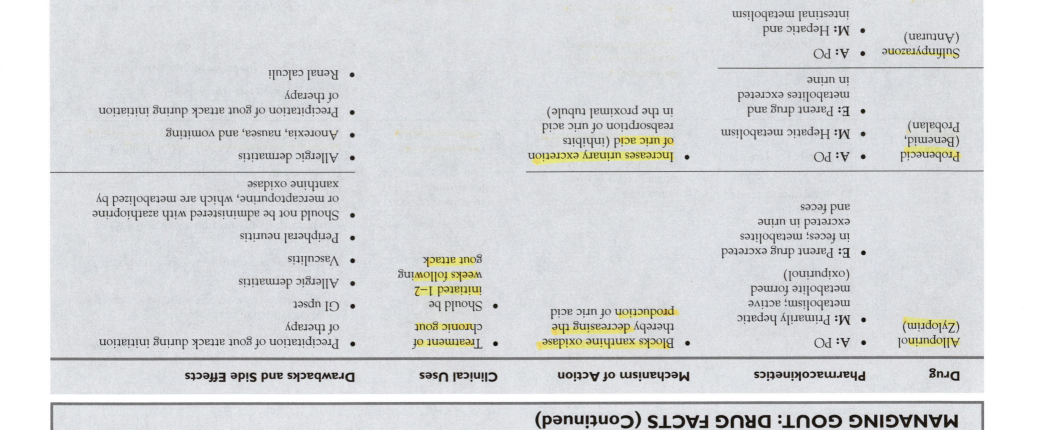

Drug	Pharmacokinetics	Mechanism of Action	Clinical Uses	Drawbacks and Side Effects
Allopurinol (Zyloprim)	• A: PO • M: Primarily hepatic metabolism; active metabolite formed (oxipurinol) • E: Parent drug excreted in feces; metabolites excreted in urine and feces	• Blocks xanthine oxidase thereby decreasing the production of uric acid	• Treatment of chronic gout • Should be initiated 1–2 weeks following gout attack	• Precipitation of gout attack during initiation of therapy • GI upset • Allergic dermatitis • Vasculitis • Peripheral neuritis • Should not be administered with azathioprine or mercaptopurine, which are metabolized by xanthine oxidase
Probenecid (Benemid, Probalan)	• A: PO • M: Hepatic metabolism • E: Parent drug and metabolites excreted in urine	• Increases urinary excretion of uric acid (inhibits reabsorption of uric acid in the proximal tubule)		• Allergic dermatitis • Anorexia, nausea, and vomiting • Precipitation of gout attack during initiation of therapy • Renal calculi
Sulfinpyrazone (Anturan)	• A: PO • M: Hepatic and intestinal metabolism • E: Parent drug and metabolites excreted in urine			

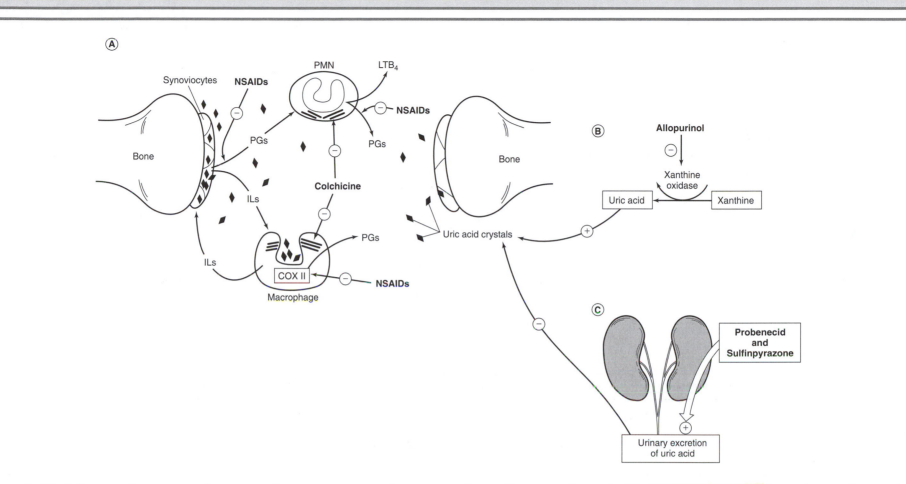

- **A:** Sites of action of some anti-inflammatory drugs in a gouty joint. Synoviocytes damaged by uric acid crystals release prostaglandins (PGs), interleukins (ILs), and other mediators of inflammation. Polymorphonuclear leukocytes (PMNs), macrophages, and other inflammatory cells enter the joint and also release inflammatory substances, including leukotrienes (eg, LTB₄), that attract additional inflammatory cells. Colchicine acts on microtubules in the inflammatory cells. NSAIDs act on COX-2 in all of the cells of the joint.
- **B:** Allopurinol decreases the production of uric acid by inhibiting xanthine oxidase.
- **C:** Probenecid and sulfinpyrazone increase the urinary excretion of uric acid by inhibiting reabsorption of uric acid in the proximal tubule.

Modified from Trevor AJ, Katzung BG, Masters SB: *Katzung & Trevor's Pharmacology Examination & Board Review*, 6th ed. Originally published by Appleton & Lange. © 2002 by the McGraw-Hill Companies, Inc.

III. Pain Relievers

CLASSIFICATION OF ANALGESICS

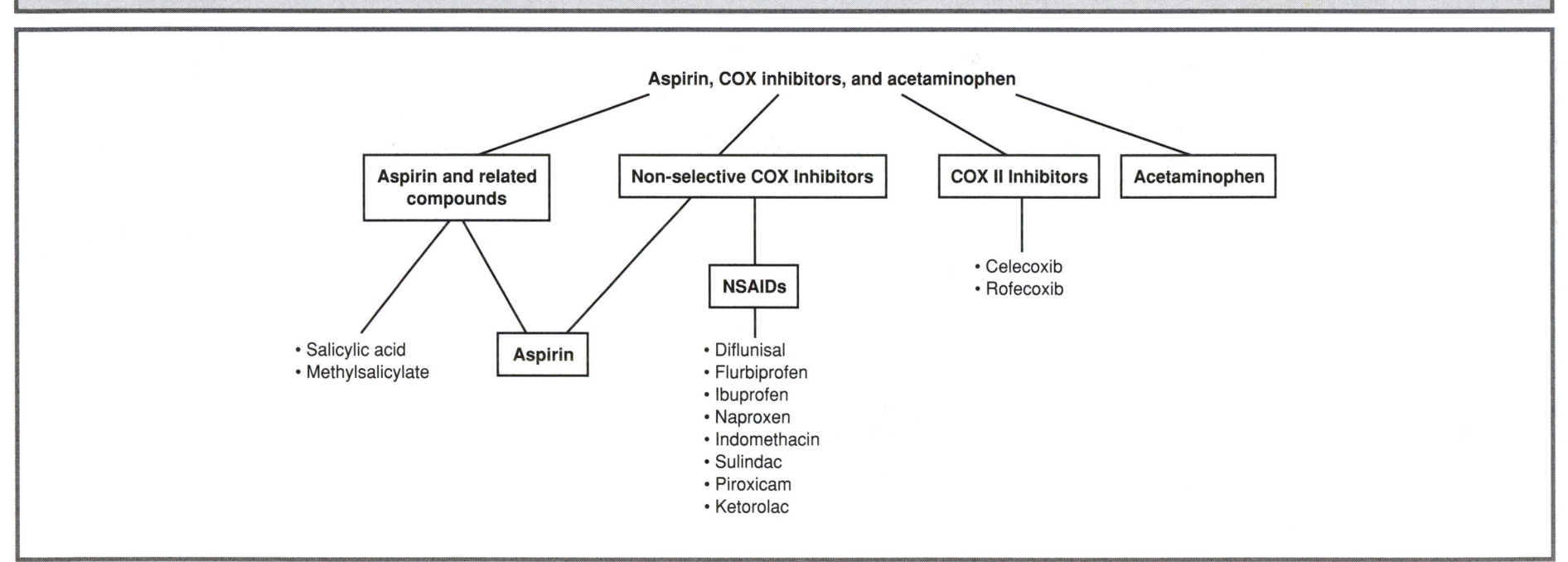

Drug	Pharmacokinetics	Clinical Uses	Drawbacks and Side Effects
Aspirin (Bayer Aspirin)	• **A:** PO and rectal • **M:** Hydrolyzed in liver, GI tract, and plasma; then further hepatic metabolism • **E:** Metabolites excreted in urine	• Fever • Mild to moderate pain relief • Inflammation and pain associated with such disorders as RA and OA • Prophylaxis for thromboembolic events (eg, CVA, MI) because of its action as a platelet aggregate inhibitor	• Contraindicated in children with viral infections • Gastritis • Increased bleeding time • Hypersensitivity • Salicylate poisoning (symptoms include agitation, convulsions, dizziness, drowsiness, fever, hallucinations, nausea, respiratory distress, tinnitus, and vomiting)
Salicylic acid	• **A:** Topical	• Acne • Dandruff • Seborrheic dermatitis • Psoriasis • Wart removal	• Skin irritation • Skin erosion • Salicylate poisoning
Methyl-salicylate (Ben-Gay)		• Topical analgesic (draws blood flow to ease myalgias)	• Salicylate poisoning (an especially potent salicylate preparation)
Acetaminophen (Tylenol)	• **A:** PO, rectal • **M:** Hepatic metabolism • **E:** Parent drug and metabolites excreted in urine	• Mild to moderate pain relief • Fever • Viral infections in children or persons with aspirin intolerance	• Few side effects • Overdose causes hepatotoxicity due to formation of reactive intermediate, N-acetyl benzoquinone imine • Treatment of overdose by N-acetylcysteine (NAC)

Continued

ASPIRIN AND RELATED COMPOUNDS, ACETAMINOPHEN, AND COX INHIBITORS (Continued)

Drug	Pharmacokinetics	Clinical Uses	Drawbacks and Side Effects
COX-2 Inhibitors			
Celecoxib (Celebrex)	• **A:** PO • **M:** Hepatic metabolism by P450 enzymes • **E:** Metabolites excreted in feces and urine	• Inflammation and pain associated with such disorders as RA and OA • Dysmenorrhea • Mild to moderate pain relief • Adjunct for reducing the number of colonic polyps in adults with familial adenomatous polyposis	• GI side effects (gastritis, GI bleeding, and ulceration) • Edema • Skin rash • Bronchitis
Rofecoxib (Vioxx)	• **A:** PO • **M:** Hepatic metabolism (P450 enzymes play a minor role) • **E:** Metabolites excreted in urine; parent drug excreted in feces	• Mild to moderate pain relief • Dysmenorrhea • Inflammation and pain associated with such disorders as RA and OA	

NONSTEROIDAL ANTI-INFLAMMATORY DRUGS

Drug	Pharmacokinetics	Clinical Uses	Side Effects
Diflunisal (Dolobid)	• **A:** PO • **M:** Hepatic metabolism • **E:** Metabolites excreted in urine	• Mild to moderate pain relief • Inflammation and pain associated with such disorders as RA and OA	• GI effects (bleeding, irritation, and ulceration) • Renal effects (dysuria, interstitial nephritis, and renal failure) • CNS effects (headache, dizziness) • Hepatic effects (jaundice, cholestatic hepatitis) • Skin effects (rash, pruritus) • Hematologic effects (thrombocytopenia, leukopenia) • Tinnitus • Blurry vision • Peripheral edema
Flurbiprofen (Ansaid)	• **A:** PO and ophthalmic • **M:** Hepatic metabolism • **E:** Parent drug and metabolites excreted in urine	• Inhibition of intraoperative miosis • Inflammation and pain associated with such disorders as RA and OA	
Ibuprofen (Motrin, Advil, and others)	• **A:** PO • **M:** Hepatic metabolism • **E:** Parent drug and metabolites excreted in urine and feces	• Mild to moderate pain relief • Treatment of pericarditis • Inflammation and pain associated with such disorders as RA and OA • Fever	
Naproxen (Naprosyn)	• **A:** PO • **M:** Hepatic metabolism • **E:** Metabolites excreted in urine	• Inflammation and pain associated with such disorders as RA and OA • Dysmenorrhea • Fever	

Continued

NONSTEROIDAL ANTI-INFLAMMATORY DRUGS (Continued)

Drug	Pharmacokinetics	Clinical Uses	Side Effects
Indomethacin (Indocin)	• **A:** PO, IV, or rectal • **M:** Hepatic metabolism • **E:** Parent drug and metabolites excreted in urine	• Inflammation and pain associated with such disorders as RA, OA, gout, and ankylosing spondylitis • Closure of patent ductus arteriosus (IV form) • Treatment of pericarditis • Dysmenorrhea • Fever • Treatment of shoulder and arm injuries (bursitis, tendinitis)	
Sulindac (Clinoril)	• **A:** PO • **M:** Prodrug that undergoes hepatic metabolism to active metabolite • **E:** Parent drug and metabolites excreted in urine and feces	• Treatment of shoulder and arm injuries (bursitis, tendinitis) • Inflammation and pain associated with such disorders as RA, OA, gout, and ankylosing spondylitis	
Piroxicam (Feldene)	• **A:** PO • **M:** Hepatic metabolism • **E:** Parent drug and metabolites excreted in urine and feces	• Inflammation and pain associated with such disorders as RA, OA, gout, and ankylosing spondylitis • Dysmenorrhea	
Ketorolac (Toradol)	• **A:** PO, IM, and IV • **M:** Hepatic metabolism • **E:** Parent drug and metabolites excreted in urine and feces	• Moderate to severe pain (eg, postoperative pain)	

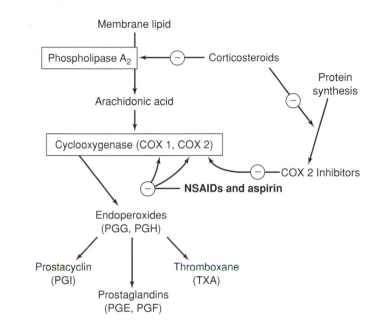

- Aspirin and NSAIDs function via inhibition of COX, which produces prostaglandin.

- COX-2 inhibitors function by inhibiting an inducible isoform of this enzyme (allows for baseline enzyme function to be maintained).

- Acetaminophen's mechanism of action remains unknown.

- Corticosteroids inhibit protein synthesis and so indirectly inhibit COX.

IV. H₁ Blockers

CLASSIFICATION OF H₁ BLOCKERS

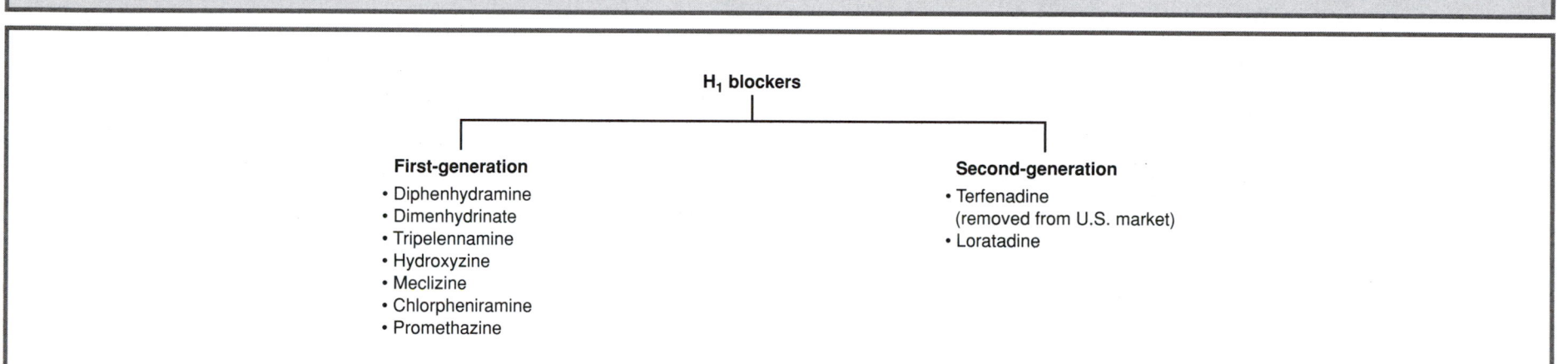

H₁ blockers

First-generation
- Diphenhydramine
- Dimenhydrinate
- Tripelennamine
- Hydroxyzine
- Meclizine
- Chlorpheniramine
- Promethazine

Second-generation
- Terfenadine
  (removed from U.S. market)
- Loratadine

FIRST- AND SECOND-GENERATION H₁ BLOCKERS

Drug	Pharmacokinetics	Mechanism of Action	Clinical Uses	Side Effects
First-Generation H₁ Blocker				
Diphenhydramine (Benadryl)	• **A:** PO, IM, IV • **M:** Metabolized by hepatic P450 enzymes • **E:** Parent drug and metabolites excreted in urine	• Compete with histamine at H₁ receptors (prevents the action of histamine) • Anticholinergic side effects also result in drying of nasal stuffiness	• Allergic reactions associated with histamine release (eg, pruritus associated with transfusions, urticaria, nasal congestion) • Motion sickness	• Sedation (more pronounced in diphenhydramine, hydroxyzine, dimenhydrinate, and tripelennamine) • Orthostatic hypotension due to α-blocker action • Anticholinergic side effects (more pronounced in diphenhydramine, dimenhydrinate, and tripelennamine)
Dimenhydrinate (Dramamine)			• Motion sickness	
Tripelennamine (Triplen, Pelamine)	• **A:** PO (hydroxyzine also available in IM form) • **M:** Metabolized by hepatic P450 enzymes • **E:** Metabolites excreted in urine		• Allergic reactions associated with histamine release (eg, nasal congestion)	
Hydroxyzine (Atarax, Vistaril)			• Allergic reactions associated with histamine release (eg, nasal congestion) • Management of acutely agitated patient	
Meclizine (Antivert)			• Motion sickness • Diseases associated with vertigo	
Chlorpheniramine (Chlor-Trimeton)			• Allergic reactions associated with histamine release (eg, nasal congestion)	

Continued

FIRST- AND SECOND-GENERATION H₁ BLOCKERS (Continued)

Drug	Pharmacokinetics	Mechanism of Action	Clinical Uses	Side Effects
Promethazine (Phenergan)	• **A:** PO, IM, IV, and rectal • **M:** Metabolized by hepatic P450 enzymes • **E:** Metabolites excreted in urine and feces		• Motion sickness • Antiemetic	
Second-Generation H₁ Blocker				
Terfenadine (Seldane)	• **A:** PO • **M:** Metabolized by hepatic P450 enzymes • **E:** Metabolites excreted in feces	• Same as above • Less sedating than first-generation	• Allergic reactions associated with histamine release (eg, nasal congestion)	• Arrhythmias (the reason why this drug has been removed from the US market) • Tremors • Headache • Rash
Loratadine (Claritin)			• Allergic reactions associated with histamine release (eg, nasal congestion)	• Tremors • Headache • Rash

CHAPTER 13
TOXICOLOGY

TERMS TO LEARN

Neutropenia	Decrease in number of neutrophils in the blood.
Paresthesias	An abnormal touch sensation (such as burning or prickling) often without external stimulus.
Systemic Lupus Erythematous	Autoimmune disorder typically seen in women; characterized by fever, polyarthritis, serositis, endocarditis, and skin rash.
Wilson's Disease	Defect in copper metabolism; leads to hepatic failure, tremor, and psychosis.

I. Managing Poisonings

TREATING SPECIFIC POISONS

Drug	Poison(s)	Mechanism of Action
N-Acetylcysteine / NAC (Mucomyst)	• Acetaminophen	• Glutathione analog that acts as a glutathione surrogate preventing the formation and accumulation of a toxic metabolite
Flumazenil (Romazicon)	• Benzodiazepines	• Direct benzodiazepine antagonist
Oxygen	• Carbon monoxide	• Competitive inhibitor with carbon monoxide for binding sites on hemoglobin
Amyl nitrite	• Cyanide	• Converts Hb to methemoglobin, which competes with cyanide for cytochrome oxidase
Sodium thiosulfate		• Converts cyanide to less toxic thiocyanate
Digoxin-specific antibodies (Digibind)	• Digoxin • Digitoxin	• Antibodies that bind excess digoxin/digitoxin creating a complex that is excreted by the kidneys
Fomepizole (Antizol)	• Methanol	• Competitive inhibitor of alcohol dehydrogenase
Ethanol	• Ethylene glycol	
Physostigmine (Antilirium, Eserine)	• Muscarinic antagonists	• Reversible inhibitor of acetylcholinesterase • Results in increased Ach to counteract muscarinic antagonism
Naloxone (Narcan)	• Opiates	• Opiate antagonist
Atropine	• Organophosphates • Carbamates • Anticholinesterases	• Muscarinic antagonist • Prevents muscarinic overactivity caused by inhibition of acetylcholinesterase
Pralidoxime (2-PAM)	• Organophosphates	• Reactivates acetylcholinesterase by cleaving the bond between the enzyme and the organophosphate • Reverses Ach overstimulation at both nicotinic and muscarinic receptors

II. Chelators

CHELATORS: DRUG FACTS

Drug	Pharmacokinetics	Clinical Uses	Side Effects
Dimercaprol/BAL	• **A:** IM • **M:** 50% rapidly metabolized to inactive metabolites • **E:** 50% chelated compound excreted in urine and feces	• Arsenic • Gold • Lead • Mercury • Sulfhydryl (–SH) group (good chelators of heavy metals)	• Transient hypertension • Tachycardia • Headache • Abdominal pain, nausea and vomiting • Paresthesias • Fevers, especially in children
Succimer/DMSA (Chemet)	• **A:** PO; variable absorption • **E:** Absorbed portion excreted unchanged in urine	• Lead • Arsenic • Mercury	• CNS effects • Elevation of liver enzymes • GI distress (nausea, vomiting, diarrhea) • Neutropenia • Skin rash
Edetate calcium disodium/ EDTA (Calcium Disodium Versenate)	• **A:** IM and IV • **E:** Unchanged in urine	• All heavy metals, especially lead	• Calcium disodium salt form prevents hypocalcemia • Hypotension • Nausea and vomiting • Nephrotoxicity • Systemic febrile reactions

| Penicillamine (Cuprimine) | • A: PO
• E: Unchanged in urine | • Arsenic
• Gold
• Lead
• Copper
• Treatment of Wilson's disease | • Nephrotoxicity with proteinuria
• Pancytopenia
• Autoimmune dysfunction, including systemic lupus erythematosus and hemolytic anemia |
| Deferoxamine (Desferel) | • A: IM or IV
• E: Unchanged in urine | • Iron | • Skin reactions
• Rapid IV administration may cause histamine release and hypotensive shock
• LTU associated with retinal degeneration, hepatic and renal dysfunction, and coagulopathies |

DMSA, dimercaptosuccinic acid; EDTA, ethylenediaminetetraacetic acid.

CHAPTER 14
ALTERNATIVE MEDICATIONS

TERMS TO LEARN

Beriberi	Syndrome associated with thiamine deficiency; symptoms include peripheral neuropathy with CHF (wet beriberi) or without CHF (dry beriberi).
Cheilosis	Noninflammatory condition of the lips; symptoms include chapping and fissuring.
Glossitis	Inflammation of the tongue.
Megaloblastic Anemia	Low blood count with a predominant number of megaloblasts in the bone marrow (enlarged cells); seen in patients with B_{12} deficiency.
Papilledema	Swelling around the optic nerve caused by pressure on the nerve by a tumor or increased intracranial pressure.
Pellagra	Syndrome associated with insufficient niacin; symptoms include dermatitis, diarrhea, dementia, and death.
Torticollis	Excessive tone in the muscles of the neck.
Xerosis	Dryness of the skin, conjunctiva, or mucous membranes.

I. Herbal Preparations

HERBAL REMEDIES: DRUG FACTS

Herb	Clinical Effects	Adverse Effects	Drug Interactions and Precautions
Clinical effects of these herbs are not based on evidence in all cases. Because herbal medications are not regulated by the FDA, their presence on the USMLE is negligible; however, they might be covered in a pharmacology course.			
Capsicum/Cayenne	• Gastroprotective agent against mucosal injury caused by aspirin • Topical treatment of pain associated with neuralgia, RA, and OA	• Stinging or burning at application site • Hypercoagulation • Hypersensitivity reactions	• Avoid contact with eyes or genitalia • Decreases bioavailability of aspirin and salicylic acid • Limit use to 2 days every 2 weeks
Cascara sagrada	• Treatment of constipation	• Arrhythmias • Neuropathies	• Thiazide diuretics, antiarrhythmics, cardiac glycosides, and indomethacin • Bowel obstruction, IBD, or abdominal pain of unknown origin
Echinacea	• Decreases duration and intensity of cold symptoms via anti-inflammatory and immunostimulating mechanisms • Treatment of UTIs • Treatment of wounds and burns	• Dizziness • GI upset • Headache • Unpleasant taste	• Immunosuppressant medications • Immunodeficiency syndromes, autoimmune disorders, or TB • Should not be taken for more than 8 weeks
Feverfew	• Decreases frequency and severity of migraine headaches	• Allergic dermatitis • GI upset • Rebound headaches	• Anticoagulants and antiplatelet drugs • May inhibit platelet aggregation

Continued

HERBAL REMEDIES: DRUG FACTS (Continued)

Herb	Clinical Effects	Adverse Effects	Drug Interactions and Precautions
Garlic	• Treatment of hyperlipidemia • Treatment of arteriosclerosis • Treatment of hypertension	• Allergic reactions • Fatigue • GI upset • Headache	• Anticoagulants and antiplatelet drugs • May inhibit platelet aggregation
Ginkgo	• Treatment of cognitive impairment associated with early Alzheimer's disease • Treatment of the symptoms of intermittent claudication • Treatment of vertigo (vascular origin) • Treatment of tinnitus (vascular origin)	• Allergic skin reactions • Bleeding • GI upset • Hypersensitivity reactions • Increased risk for spontaneous intracranial hemorrhage	• Anticoagulants and antiplatelet drugs • May inhibit platelet aggregation • Intracranial hemorrhage
Ginseng	• Treatment of fatigue and debility • May improve mental and physical performance	• Hypertension • Insomnia • Mastalgia • Nervousness • Vaginal bleeding	• Psychiatric medications (eg, MAO inhibitors), loop diuretics, anticoagulants, or diabetes medications
Goldenseal	• External antiseptic • Treatment of diarrhea caused by numerous GI pathogens • Treatment of trachoma • Treatment of gastric ulcers • Treatment of gallbladder disease	• GI disorders associated with LTU	• Contraindicated in patients with G6PD deficiency • May antagonize the action of heparin

Kava	• Treatment of chronic anxiety states	• Ataxia • Drowsiness • Hepatotoxicity • Sedation • Skin rash • Torticollis	• Barbiturates, alcohol, DA agonists or antagonists • Endogenous depression (increases risk of suicide)
Ma-huang (Ephedra)	• Treatment of cough and bronchitis (bronchodilator) • CNS stimulant • Diet aid	• Arrhythmias • CVA • Headache • Hypertension • Insomnia • MI • Nervousness • Tremor • Seizures	• Cardiac glycosides, Guanethidine, MAO inhibitors, or other CNS stimulants
Milk thistle	• Treatment of liver and gallbladder disorders • Treatment of dyspepsia • Improves hepatic function in viral hepatitis • Antidote to *Amanita* mushroom poisoning (hepatotoxicity)	• GI upset (nausea, diarrhea, vomiting, abdominal cramping)	• Using milk thistle with typical antipsychotics can alter lipid peroxidation
Saw palmetto	• Improves urinary symptoms associated with BPH (no change in gland size) • Treatment of irritable bladder	• Decreased libido • GI upset • Headache • Hypertension	• Hormones or hormone-like medications • May possess androgenic, estrogenic, and α-blocking effects

Continued

HERBAL REMEDIES: DRUG FACTS (Continued)

Herb	Clinical Effects	Adverse Effects	Drug Interactions and Precautions
St. John's wort	• Treatment of mild to moderate depression • Promotes healing of burns and wounds	• Allergic reactions • Confusion • Dizziness • Dry mouth • Fatigue • GI upset • Photosensitivity	• Antidepressants, such as SSRIs and MAO inhibitors; drugs that cause photosensitivity, such as tetracycline; numerous other drug interactions due to induction of P450 enzymes • Decreases absorption of iron
Valerian	• Treatment of nervousness • Treatment of insomnia	• GI upset	• CNS depressants (such as barbiturates, benzodiazepines, or alcohol) because it has an additive CNS depressive effect
Yohimbe bark	• Sympatholytic agent • Mydriatic agent • Treatment of impotence with vascular or psychogenic origin	• Dizziness • Headache • Hypertension • Tachycardia	• OTC stimulants, alcohol, antidepressants, or antihypertensives • Liver or kidney diseases

Physicians Desk Reference for Herbal Medicines, 2nd ed.

II. Vitamins

WATER SOLUBLE AND FAT SOLUBLE VITAMINS

Water Soluble Vitamins	Fat Soluble Vitamins
B_1 (Thiamine)	A
B_2 (Riboflavin)	D
B_3 (Niacin)	E
B_5 (Pantothenic acid)	K
B_6 (Pyridoxine)	
B_{12}	
Biotin	
Folic acid	
C	

☞ Water Soluble Vitamins: "See–C– the Bs drinking water" because biotin and folic acid are considered to be B-complex vitamins.

ADEK can be used to remember the fat-soluble vitamins; each letter represents one of the vitamins.

To remember which vitamin is B_1, B_2, or B_3, use the word **TRaiN**. The letters correspond to **t**hiamine (B_1), **r**iboflavin (B_2), and **n**iacin (B_3). All B vitamins function as coenzymes.

VITAMINS: DRUG FACTS

Vitamin	Deficiency	Overdose
Vitamin A*	• Xerosis (dry skin) • Night blindness • Blindness (most common type of preventable blindness in children)	• Acute toxicity (increased intracranial pressure, headaches, and papilledema) • Alopecia • Arthralgia • Hepatosplenomegaly
Vitamin B$_1$ (Thiamine)	• Beriberi (visual disturbances, paralysis, paresthesias of lower extremities, psychosis, and CHF) • Wernicke-Korsakoff syndrome	• None
Vitamin B$_2$ (Riboflavin)	• Mild symptoms (chelosis, corneal vascularization, angular stomatitis)	• None documented • Possible increase in the risk of stomach cancer
Vitamin B$_3$ (Niacin)	• Pellagra (diarrhea, dermatitis, and dementia)	• Facial flushing • Hyperuricemia • Liver dysfunction • Pruritus
Vitamin B$_5$ (Pantothenic acid)	• Alopecia • Dermatitis • GI upset	• None
Vitamin B$_6$ (Pyridoxine)	• Angular stomatitis • Dermatitis • Glossitis • Peripheral neuropathy • Often associated with isoniazid therapy	• Sensory neuropathy

Vitamin B$_{12}$	• Megaloblastic anemia • Glossitis • Neurologic disorders	• None
Biotin	• Dermatitis • Enteritis	• None
Folic Acid	• Neural tube defects • Megaloblastic anemia	• None
Vitamin C (Ascorbic acid)	• Scurvy	• GI upset • Kidney stones
Vitamin D*	• Ricket's disease (in children) • Osteomalacia (in adults) • Hypocalcemia	• Hypercalcemia • Mental and growth retardation in children • Kidney failure • Death
Vitamin E*	• Increased fragility of erythrocytes • Peripheral neuropathy (motor and sensory)	• Diarrhea • Fatigue • Kidney stones • Nausea
Vitamin K*	• Bleeding disorders	• Rash • Itching

*Fat soluble vitamins.

INDEX

B

Bacitracin (Baciguent, Neosporin), 33
Baclofen (Lioresal), 121, 166
Barbiturates
    methohexital (Brevital), 176
    pentobarbital (Nembutal), 145
    phenobarbital, 121, 145, 148
    secobarbital (Seconal), 145
    thiopental (Pentothal), 145, 176
Beclomethasone (Vancenase), 246
Benazepril (Lotensin), 208
Benzocaine (Americaine), 170
Benzodiazepines
    alprazolam (Xanax), 143
    diazepam (Valium), 142
    estazolam (ProSom), 143
    flurazepam (Dalmane), 142
    lorazepam (Ativan), 143
    midazolam (Versed), 176
    oxazepam, 144
    quazepam (Doral), 143
    temazepam (Restoril), 144
    triazolam (Halcion), 144
Benzonatate (Tessalon), 242
Benztropine (Cogentin), 134
Beriberi, definition of, 352
β-blockers, 199
    acebutolol (Sectral), 98
    atenolol (Tenormin), 98
    carvedilol (Coreg), 99, 216
    esmolol (Brevibloc), 98
    labetalol (Normodyne, Trandate), 99, 216
    metoprolol (Lopressor, Toprol), 98, 216
    nadolol (Corgard), 98
    pindolol (Viskin), 98
    propranolol (Inderal), 99, 163, 191, 209, 216

sotalol (Betapace), 99, 199
timolol (Blocadren, Timoptic), 99, 103
β-lactamase–resistant penicillins
    cloxacillin (Tegopen), 17, 20
    methicillin (Staphcillin), 17, 20
    nafcillin (Nallpen), 17, 20
    oxacillin (Bactocill), 17, 20
β_2-adrenergic agonists
    albuterol (Proventil, Ventolin), 244
    formoterol (Foradil), 245
    isoetharine, 244
    isoproterenol (Isuprel), 244
    metaproterenol (Alupent, Metaprel), 244
    salmeterol (Serevent), 245
    terbutaline (Brethine), 245
Betaxolol (Betoptic), 103
Bethanechol (Urecholine, Duvoid, Urabeth), 83
Bile acid sequestrants
    cholestipol (Cholestid), 228
    cholestyramine (Questran), 228
Binding, 9
Bioavailability, definition of, 2
Biotin, 359
Biphosphonates
    alendronate (Foramax), 273
    etidronate (Didronel), 274
    pamidronate (Aredia), 274
    risedronate (Actonel), 274
Bismuth-based triple therapy, 256
Bismuth subsalicylate (Pepto Bismol), 254
Bitolterol (Tornolate), 93
Blackwater fever, definition of, 15
Bleomycin (Blenoxane), 306
Blepharospasm, definition of, 131
Blood dyscrasias, definition of, 150
Blood-to-gas partition coefficient (B/G coefficient), definition of, 131
Botulinium toxin (BoTox), 167

Bretylium (Bretylol), 200
Brimonidine (Alphagan), 102
Bromocriptine (Parlodel), 137, 266
Buccal adminstration route, 9
Bumetanide (Bumex), 223
Bupivacaine (Marcaine), 171
Buprenorphine (Buprenex), 159
Bupropion (Wellbutrin), 115
Buspirone (Buspar), 146
Busulfan (Myleran, Busulfex), 300
Butorphanol (Stadol), 159
Butyrophenones
    droperidol (Inapsine), 109
    haloperidol (Haldol), 109

C

Cabergoline (Dostinex), 266
Caffeine, 126
Caffeine and ergotamine (Cafergot), 161
CAI (carbonic acid inhibitor) diuretic
    acetazolamide (Diamox), 225
Calcium carbonate, 252
Calcium channel blockers
    diltiazem (Cardizem, Dilacor), 190, 200, 219
    nifedipine (Adalat, Procardia), 191, 219
    verapamil (Calan, Isoptin), 164, 190, 200, 219
Calcium levels, drugs affecting
    antineoplastic agent
        plicamycin (Mithracin), 275
    biphosphonates
        alendronate (Foramax), 273
        etidronate (Didronel), 274
        pamidronate (Aredia), 274
        risedronate (Actonel), 274
    clinical uses, 276
    dental prophylaxis
        sodium fluoride (Fluoritab), 275